Food Intolerance

FOOD SAFETY SERIES

General Series Editors
J. Edelman *London, UK*
S. Miller *Texas, USA*

Series Editor — Microbiology
T. Roberts *Reading, UK*

Editorial Board
D. Conning *London, UK*
D. Georgala *Reading, UK*
J. Houtvast *Wageningen, The Netherlands*
C. Mercier *Paris, France*
E. Widdowson *Cambridge, UK*

Forthcoming Titles
Immunoassays for Food-poisoning
Bacteria and Bacterial Toxins
G. Wyatt

The *Staphylococci* and their Toxins
M. Bergdoll

The *Aeromonas* Group as a Foodborne Pathogen
S. Palumbo and F. Busta

Food Preservation
G. Gould

Fibre and Complex Carbohydrates
I. Johnson and D. Southgate

Food Intolerance

Maurice H. Lessof

Emeritus Professor of Medicine
United Medical and Dental Schools
Guy's and St Thomas's Hospitals

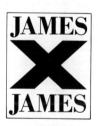

CHAPMAN & HALL
London · Glasgow · New York · Tokyo · Melbourne · Madras

Co-published by James & James (Science Publishers) Ltd, 5 Castle Road, London NW1 8PR, UK and Chapman & Hall, 2–6 Boundary Row, London SE1 8HN, UK

Chapman & Hall, 2–6 Boundary Row, London SE1 8HN, UK

Blackie Academic & Professional, Wester Cleddens Road, Bishopbriggs, Glasgow G64 2NZ, UK

Van Nostrand Reinhold Inc., 115 5th Avenue, New York NY10003, USA

Chapman & Hall Japan, Thomson Publishing Japan, Hirakawacho Nemoto Building, 6F, 1-7-11 Hirakawa-cho, Chiyoda-ku, Tokyo 102, Japan

Chapman & Hall Australia, Thomas Nelson Australia, 102 Dodds Street, South Melbourne, Victoria 3205, Australia

Chapman & Hall India, R. Seshadri, 32 Second Main Road, CIT East, Madras 600 035, India

First edition 1992
© 1992 M. H. Lessof

Typeset in 12/13pt Garamond 3 by Columns of Reading Ltd
Printed in Great Britain

ISBN 0 412 448505 ✓

A catalogue record for this book is available from the British Library

Library of Congress Cataloging-in-Publication data available

For Leila

Contents

Series introduction   ix

1   Nutrition in the modern world   1
    1.1   Escape from malnutrition and contaminated food   1
    1.2   Food problems of the affluent society   2
       1.2.1   Lifestyle, diet and disease   3
    1.3   What is a healthy diet?   6
    1.4   Food as a focus of anxieties   8
       1.4.1   'Fast foods' and 'E' numbers   9
       1.4.2   Food ingredients: fibre   11
       1.4.3   The 'saccharine' diseases   13
    1.5   Food and coronary artery disease   14
       1.5.1   Salt and high blood pressure   15
    1.6   Back to nature?   16
    1.7   Conclusion   17

2   Food intolerance and attitudes to food   18
    2.1   Definitions   18
    2.2   Epidemiology   20
    2.3   Eating habits   22
    2.4   The eating disorders   24
       2.4.1   Food faddism   24
       2.4.2   Anorexia, bulimia and obesity   25

	2.4.3	Psychiatric illness and food	28
	2.4.4	Childhood hyperactivity: food-related or yet another 'attitude'?	29
	2.5	Conclusion	34

3	Food and alternative medicine	35
	3.1	Ecology and the protest movement	35
		3.1.1 The problems of pollution	36
	3.2	Food and the counterrevolution	39
		3.2.1 The total allergy syndrome	41
		3.2.2 Unorthodox diagnosis and treatment	42
	3.3	Alternative medical practice and the patient	47
		3.3.1 Diagnoses which can be missed	49
	3.4	Conclusion	51

4	Physiology of digestion	52
	4.1	Basic functions of the gut	52
		4.1.1 Role of the digestive enzymes	56
		4.1.2 Role of bile	56
	4.2	Mucosal immunity	58
		4.2.1 Amplifying mechanisms	65
		4.2.2 Immune responses to ingested substances	65
		4.2.3 Antigenic foods	66
		4.2.4 Biogenic Amines	67
	4.3	Disorders of intestinal motility	70
	4.4	Conclusion	71

5	Mechanisms of food intolerance	73
	5.1	Immune responses provoked by food	74
		5.1.1 Type 1 reactions	74
		5.1.2 Type 2 reactions	76
		5.1.3 Type 3 reactions	77
		5.1.4 Type 4 reactions	78
	5.2	How much is immunological?	78
	5.3	Pseudoallergic mechanisms	81
		5.3.1 Toxic effects	81
		5.3.2 Pharmacological effects	81
		5.3.3 Enzyme defects	81

| | 5.3.4 | Complex mechanisms | 85 |
| 5.4 | | Conclusion | 85 |

6		Clinical manifestations	87
	6.1	Establishing the diagnosis	87
		6.1.1 Validity of tests	87
	6.2	Food intolerance in childhood	90
		6.2.1 Incidence	91
		6.2.2 Infantile eczema	95
		6.2.3 Childhood asthma	96
		6.2.4 Other childhood symptoms	98
	6.3	Reactions in older children and adults	98
		6.3.1 Food antigens and cross-reactions	99
		6.3.2 Clinical features	101
		6.3.3 Diagnosis of food-induced asthma	108
		6.3.4 Headache, migraine and neurological symptoms	109
		6.3.5 The joints	112
		6.3.6 The kidney	114
		6.3.7 The blood	114
	6.4	Occupational reactions to food	115
		6.4.1 Management of adverse reactions	117
	6.5	Conclusion	122

7		Food additives	123
	7.1	What are they?	123
	7.2	How did the use of additives develop?	127
	7.3	Regulations on food additives	128
	7.4	Examples of additives in current use	129
	7.5	Do additives cause unpleasant reactions	131
		7.5.1 Sulphites	131
		7.5.2 Benzoates and parabens	133
		7.5.3 Coal-tar dyes	134
		7.5.4 Monosodium glutamate	134
		7.5.5 Aspartame	135
		7.5.6 Other additives	135
		7.5.7 Regulating additive usage	136
	7.6	Confirming clinical suspicions	137
		7.6.1 Estimates of prevalence	138
	7.7	Do we need them?	139
	7.8	Conclusion	140

8 Cow's milk and some alternatives   142
   8.1   Allergens of cow's milk   143
   8.2   Alternatives to cow's milk   144
   8.3   Cow's milk protein intolerance: prevention,
         treatment and research   146
         8.3.1   The case for hydrolysates   147
   8.4   Alternative approaches to milk processing   148
         8.4.1   Milk homogenization   148
         8.4.2   Effects of heat-processing   149
         8.4.3   Milk fermentation and cheese-ripening   150
         8.4.4   Hyposensitizing milk formulas   151
   8.5   Conclusion   153

9 Gluten sensitivity and coeliac disease   154
   9.1   Coeliac disease and prolamin toxicity   155
   9.2   Nature of gluten sensitivity   157
         9.2.1   Racial and geographical prevalence   159
         9.2.2   Clinical features   160
         9.2.3   Unusual presentations   162
         9.2.4   Mucosal damage and its effect on symptoms   164
   9.3   Dietary management   166
   9.4   Conclusion   166

10   The patient's dilemma   168
   10.1   Initiating a diet   169
   10.2   Patient self-help groups   170
   10.3   Maternal problems   172
   10.4   Dietary errors   173
   10.5   The doctor-patient relationship   174
   10.6   Diagnostic tests   175
   10.7   The need for better information   177
   10.8   Conclusion   179

Glossary   180

References   187

Index   204

Series Introduction

Consumer safety has become a central issue of the food supply system in most countries. It encompasses a large number of interacting scientific and technological matters, such as agricultural practice, microbiology, chemistry, food technology, processing, handling and packaging. The techniques used in understanding and controlling contaminants and toxicity range from the most sophisticated scientific laboratory methods, through industrial engineering science to simple logical rules implemented in the kitchen.

The problems of food safety, however, spread far beyond those directly occupied in food production. Public interest and concern has become acute in recent years, alerting a wide spectrum of specialists in research, education and public affairs.

This series aims to present timely volumes covering all aspects of the subject. They will be up-to-date, specialist reviews written by acknowledged experts in their fields of research to express each author's own viewpoint. The readership is intended to be wide and international, and the style to be comprehensible to non-specialists, albeit professionals.

The series will be of interest to food scientists and technologists working in industry, universities, polytechnics and government institutes; legislators and regulators concerned with the food supply; and specialists in agriculture, engineering, health care and consumer affairs.

Perhaps no aspect of food safety has attracted more attention than people's reaction to food itself. Intolerance by some individuals to specific foods or their components is well documented. This can range from true allergies to psychologically based aversions, and is often difficult to diagnose. Real knowledge and advice in the subject is not easy to come by. Professor Lessof, himself a distinguished medical specialist, has made an intensive study of the subject, so his book will appeal to medical practitioners and other health care workers.

But the problem impinges on the food supply system as a whole; Professor Lessof's book has been written with a view to informing not only the medical world, but agriculturalists, retailers, legislators, consumer groups and others concerned with the well-being of the public at large.

J. Edelman

CHAPTER

—1—

Nutrition in the Modern World

ESCAPE FROM MALNUTRITION AND CONTAMINATED FOOD

Many of the problems of the underdeveloped countries arise from the lack of an adequate and clean supply of food. Some of their principal health problems, therefore, relate to malnutrition and the infections transmitted by food and water. The privileged Western countries are not, however, free of difficulties. The developed West has a surfeit of food and has the means to harvest and store food in clean conditions with only a relatively low risk of contamination during storage. These countries are more likely to have to deal with the hazards of food excess than the problems of food shortage (*Macdonald, 1983*).

There are other problems caused by food in the more sophisticated communities. Infections still occur and, even when avoided, other difficulties can be caused by the deterioration of processed food during prolonged storage. There may also be risks associated with the refining or preservation of food by modern methods, including the occasional possibility of some form of food reaction or intolerance. The part played by food processing in this risk is probably small, as people who react adversely to manufactured food products are considerably fewer than those who have allergic or intolerant reactions to unprocessed food (*Young et al., 1987*).

In the West, the problem of adverse food reactions has not hitherto

1

been considered to be of particular importance compared to the problems of an ill-chosen or unbalanced diet, or the problem of overnutrition, in which more food is absorbed than can be metabolized (utilized, stored, broken down or excreted). Its importance should be kept in a proper perspective – in comparison to those nutritional disorders which are among the scourges of Western society and are most common in the obese, or in those whose diet is rich in animal fats or lacking in vegetables and complex carbohydrates.

The general public has not always seen these problems for what they are. The dangers of gluttony have provided a time-honoured theme, and the need for healthy eating and drinking habits has received some emphasis. Alongside this, however, there has been an upsurge of less informed and more sensational information about food and its hazards, often exploited by a communication industry which spreads its ideas, both good and bad, with frightening speed and with dramatic emphasis. The opinion-forming role of the media, aided by sophisticated pressure groups, has been extraordinary and, in matters of nutrition, the misinformation spread by sensation-mongers or vested-interest groups has led to considerable social problems. Information concerning food allergy and intolerance has been distorted into alarmist propaganda.

The dangers of Western food have captured the imagination of journalists, who have developed catch-phrase warnings about becoming 'allergic to the twentieth century'. There is now on offer a range of tests and treatments for remedies, both real and imagined, which have been linked to either natural or processed food. The evidence on which these claims are based deserves further consideration.

FOOD PROBLEMS OF THE AFFLUENT SOCIETY

Evolution has equipped virtually all living things with the ability to cope with fluctuations in the food supply. In the short term, a temporary excess or deficiency of food is met in humans by either a build-up or depletion of the energy stores of the body, especially in the form of fat. During longer periods of either over- or underfeeding, adaptations occur which increase or reduce the rate of energy expenditure so that, except in continuing conditions of gluttony or starvation, gross fat deposition or depletion become difficult to achieve (*Garrow & Blaza, 1982*). In the more wealthy countries, such gross changes in the fat depots are usually due to excessive food intake, allowing obesity to become the most common nutritional problem of the affluent society.

Not surprisingly, there is considerable individual variation in the effectiveness of the regulating mechanisms which control weight. Where those regulating mechanisms fail, obesity can follow even in people who eat no more – or may even eat less – than others whose weight is constant. It has been shown that energy requirements vary widely from one individual to another; consequently, a very high food intake does not always lead to fat deposition. The hazards of overnutrition and the potential damage to the joints, cardiovascular system, and metabolic processes of the body relate more closely to the degree of obesity than to the amount of food intake. Fat people tend to die younger from conditions ranging from coronary artery disease and heart failure to diabetes and chest infections. As medical insurance companies have shown, they are also more likely to develop arthritis, hernias, varicose veins, gall bladder disease and a host of other ailments. Most of the problems which they suffer in relation to food are long-term problems that are predominantly associated with excess and often correctable by lifestyle changes involving less food intake and more exercise.

There is one exception to this epidemiological hazard of the obese – obese individuals are less likely to commit suicide. It remains uncertain whether this is because overweight persons are less prone to become depressed or whether, if depressed, they are less likely to follow a course which requires physical action.

Lifestyle, Diet and Disease

By a curious analogy, the potential damage which can accrue from inappropriate lifestyle changes was well illustrated by a study not of humans, but of zoo animals. Dr Peter Wise, an endocrinologist, investigated an especially high death rate among gerbils and other small desert animals. It appeared that, in their inhospitable environment, nature had adapted the metabolism of these creatures so that they could lay down fat in their fat depots even under the most inauspicious circumstances. This metabolic adaptation, so helpful in times of hardship, proved a disaster in times of plenty as their metabolic pathways became saturated. Many animals in The London Zoo were so well fed that their fat-depositing mechanisms were overwhelmed. They developed and died of diabetes.

In humans, the problem of diabetes in the obese has long been recognized, but it is clear that not all obese subjects are equally affected. As in zoo animals, the individuals who make up a genetically diverse population may have metabolic control systems which function at different levels. Whereas one individual can become very obese without any obvious defect in glucose metabolism, another may develop non-insulin dependent diabetes when only mildly obese or not obese at all. South Asians or immigrants from the Indian subcontinent now living in Great Britain have high rates of diabetes, sometimes associated with a high blood pressure or coronary artery disease, and with a striking tendency to accumulate fat centrally in the body (*McKeigue, 1991*). The response to overnutrition and lack of physical exercise appears to differ from that of the indigenous population, and there may be evidence of insulin resistance and a disturbed metabolism of lipids.

In a human 'outbred' population, there are other consequences of overnutrition or an unhealthy diet which may vary according to the individual's genetic make-up or as a result of other environmental factors. The effects of dietary fat on the serum lipid and cholesterol concentration levels vary enormously from one person to another, depending on age, gender, physical activity, mental activity, cigarette-smoking and alcohol consumption. The dramatic fall in the prevalence of ischaemic heart disease that has taken place in the United States may be the result of a sharply reduced intake of fat, including saturated fat, and an increased emphasis on the avoidance of obesity. On the other hand, a trend towards an increase in physical exercise – for example, by jogging – and the decline in cigarette-smoking may well have also contributed to this change. The complex interaction of these different influences has been emphasized by the recent rise in deaths from cardiovascular diseases in Eastern Europe at the same time as such deaths have been falling in several Western countries and in Japan. In many instances, changes in smoking habits rather than diet could account for the decreases, but dietary factors and high standards of living could well have a protective effect and may have contributed to the remarkably low death rate in Japan, which is against the trend which might have been predicted from Japanese smoking habits.

One of the difficulties in demonstrating a link between diet and disease lies in the long latent period which may occur between the consumption of dietary substances and their consequences. In young American soldiers who were killed in Korea, a high incidence of atheroma was found, providing clear evidence that this can be laid down in substantial amounts by the age of 20 years. That does not indicate, however, that these changes are irreversible. In Norway in World War II, there was a sharp fall in the incidence of ischaemic heart disease at a time of severe food deprivation and at a time, furthermore, of great stress. It appeared that dietary deprivation was followed by a fall in the incidence of heart disease after a very short latent period, but this was increased as soon as food supplies became more normal (*Macdonald, 1983*). The reversibility of diet-related atherosclerosis has also been demonstrated more recently (*Ornish et al., 1990*).

The adverse effects of a poor or unbalanced diet are, in general, long-term effects. It is the problems of excess that have attracted most attention in Western countries, whereas the more immediate and dramatic food-induced illnesses have been considerably less important in these affluent communities. Illness caused by contaminated and infected food can nevertheless cause major outbreaks of illness or even death, especially among frail or elderly people. As a public health problem, there is always the risk of outbreaks of gastroenteritis due to poor standards of hygiene among chicken farmers or other food producers, or among food purveyors or restauranteurs. There is also the risk that food can become contaminated if it is badly stored or transported, or if, as in some recent cases, the precautionary use of preservatives is abandoned because of a rejection of modern technology and an attempt to return to what is deemed to be a more natural method of food production which avoids the use of all additives.

Less common than the problems of overnutrition, malnutrition or contaminated food are the unpleasant and occasionally serious reactions provoked by ordinary dietary items in a small minority of unusually susceptible people. These problems of food intolerance are the main subject of this volume and include specific allergic reactions to food as well as enzyme deficiencies and coeliac disease. These disorders can present in a variety of ways and mainly affect the skin, the nasal passages and lung airways, and the stomach and bowel.

WHAT IS A HEALTHY DIET?

A healthy diet requires protein foods for growth and repair, carbohydrates and fats for energy, and foods which contain adequate quantities of essential minerals and vitamins. The ideal contribution from various types of food are shown in Table 1.1. While paediatricians assert that these limits are unsuitable for growing children (*MacNair, 1991*), there is little doubt that the diet of most adults in the United Kingdom and Northern Europe contains too much fat, sugar and salt, and too little starchy food, fruit and vegetables (*James & Ralph, 1990*). The recommendations for protein are not always tabulated. It is evident that the proportion of energy derived from protein (12%) in a survey of 10–15-year-old British schoolchildren is below the 15–20% regarded as ideal in North America and in the UK, but well above the achievable level in less developed countries.

While the proportion of energy derived from protein, fat (37–38%), and carbohydrate (49–50%) has remained virtually unchanged in British schoolchildren between 1936 and 1983, the total energy intake fell by 20–30%, possibly reflecting a more sedentary

Table 1.1 Comparison between World Health Organization (WHO) dietary recommendations and current UK diet

	WHO recommendations	Current UK average
Energy (%) derived from:		
Total fat	15–< 30	35–40
Saturated fat	< 10	17
Starchy foods	45–55	28
Added sugars	< 10	17
Vegetables and fruit (g/day)	> 400	246
Dietary fibre (non-starchy polysaccharides; g/day)	20	13
Salt (g/day)	< 6	8

Modified from *James & Ralph, 1990; WHO, 1990*

lifestyle. Since 1983, there has been a new emphasis on health education together with an appreciation of the advantages of most Mediterranean diets, with a high proportion of starchy foods and a low proportion of saturated fatty acids. There can no longer be any justification for the traditional belief that starchy foods are fattening. The foods which should be reduced in quantity are not starchy foods, but those which are rich in saturated fatty acids or added sugar.

In addition to the main nutrients, a healthy diet requires adequate (but not excessive) amounts of electrolytes, trace elements (Table 1.2) and vitamins (Table 1.3), all of which have an important role in the production of enzymes or co-factors which help the metabolic processes. These substances are, in general, available in adequate amounts, but calcium and zinc may be poorly absorbed if there is a high intake of fibre or phytate. Iron is deficient in some vegetarian diets, and a lack of iodine may be a problem in some inland areas.

Vitamin deficiencies can occur more readily when the diet is unbalanced rather than grossly inadequate. An example is found in the deficiency of thiamine (vitamin B_1), most often seen in areas where most of the diet depends on unenriched white flour or rice, but also in alcoholics, who may also be deficient in other B vitamins such as riboflavin (B_2) and pyridoxine (B_6). Ascorbic acid (vitamin C) deficiency usually reflects a lack of fruit and vegetables, but requirements may be increased in response to infection or injury. Vitamin D deficiency may arise if there is a poor dietary intake, but also if there is a lack of

Table 1.2 Recommended daily adult intake of calcium, magnesium and trace elements

Calcium	600 mg (1200 mg in pregnancy and lactation)
Magnesium	280–350 mg
Iron	10 mg (12–15 mg in premenopausal women)
Zinc	12–15 mg
Manganese	2–5 mg
Copper	1.5–3 mg
Fluoride	1.5–4 mg
Iodine	0.15 mg
Chromium	0.05–0.2 mg
Selenium	0.05–0.07 mg
Molybdenum	0.075–0.25 mg

Table 1.3 Recommended daily adult intake of vitamins

Vitamin A	Retinol equivalents	750 μg
B vitamins	Thiamine	1–1.3 mg
	Riboflavin	1.6 mg
	Nicotinic acid equivalents	18 mg
	Total folate	300 μg
Vitamin C	Ascorbic acid	30 mg
Vitamin D	Cholecalciferol	None if adequate sunshine[a]
Vitamin E	Alpha-tocopherol equivalents	8–10 mg
Vitamin K	Clotting-factor precursors	70–140 μg

[a] 10 μg (400 IU) supplements for children in winter, and for housebound adults

sunshine or fat malabsorption. Conditions which reduce the absorption of fat can also reduce the absorption of vitamins A, E and K.

FOOD AS A FOCUS OF ANXIETIES

There is a great deal of difference between a reasonable interest in a healthy diet and an undue concern about the dangers of unhealthy foods, or the possibility of ill health arising from an intolerant reaction to specific foods. Much more common than the problems of food intolerance are the anxieties which are focused upon food. Food and the events associated with its preparation and provision fulfil both emotional and biological needs, and the effects of the emotions upon appetite need no emphasis. Some seek solace in food or attach a ritual importance to it. It has become the object of numerous anxieties and feelings of guilt, either in those who fear obesity or in those who are influenced by adverse publicity concerning food products. Responding to this publicity, many members of the public have become convinced that faulty industrial food preparation – in particular, the use of additives – is responsible for a wide range of insidious and ill-defined symptoms.

Adverse reactions to food have thus been blamed for causing a variety of unpleasant effects, often with little evidence to support such a claim. Many obese people who read a recent article in the London Daily Express (9 September, 1991) were told that most obesity is due to fluid retention, that most fluid retention is due to allergy, and that an £80 cytotoxic blood test could identify the foods responsible. Despite the sweeping nature of these unsubstantiated claims, the laboratory concerned received 7,000 enquiries about its method within a week. 'At last', the reporter had written, 'a scientific answer to slimmers' nightmares'.

For whatever reason, some members of the medical profession have encouraged public fears and anxieties about food safety and its ability to cause sensitivity and disease. These fears are sometimes difficult to counter, since medical diagnosis remains an imperfect science and, where symptoms remain unexplained, it may be difficult to disprove allegations that vague symptoms such as headache, insomnia, tinnitus, palpitations, breathlessness, ankle swelling, abdominal bloating, and fatigue are indeed food-related. Those who follow this argument may come to regard food as an almost universal scapegoat and blame a wide range of symptoms on an increasing number of foods. Following this theme, adverse reactions to food have also been used to explain bad behaviour in childhood, bed-wetting, learning difficulties and hyperactivity. Associations of this kind must be treated with scepticism unless they can be substantiated by objective scientific assessment.

The fashion for attributing vague symptoms to food allergy may have passed its peak. Similar symptoms have, in the past, been attributed to 'dropped organs' or visceroptosis, intestinal stasis, chronic appendicitis, vitamin deficiencies and low blood sugar but, as with the clinical ecologist's diagnosis of food allergy or candida hypersensitivity, confirmatory evidence was lacking. Without adequate methods of testing, the various rival diagnoses become a matter of opinion, but the reliance of different practitioners on totally different diagnoses to explain almost identical symptoms must inevitably raise questions as to their validity. Contradictory claims are not uncommon – for example, candidiasis of the intestine explains a vast range of symptoms, or it is rare; or food-provoked childhood hyperactivity affects over 5% of American schoolchildren, but far fewer British children on a similar diet (see Chapter 2).

'Fast Foods' and 'E' Numbers

The marketing of ready-prepared foods has become a boom industry not only in the Western hemisphere, where the fashion began, but also in Europe and other countries. This has led to concerns about the high fat content of hamburgers and other prepared foods, and about the difficulty the consumer may have in identifying the components which make up the final product. It has also led to anxieties over the safety of the food additives which are used during processing in order to give a packaged food a reasonable shelf-life, or a consistent and attractive appearance and flavour. Those who, rightly or wrongly, believe that food additives make them ill sometimes claim that the methods of high-yield farming, and the use of modern techniques of food processing and of additives to prevent deterioration in storage, have all led to serious health hazards. They believe that the very methods that were designed to achieve a secure and safe food supply for large populations have achieved their results only at the cost of danger and discomfort.

In Europe, food-labelling requirements have been introduced in order to identify the additives that are present in a particular food preparation. 'E' numbers have been given to those additives recognized by the European Community as safe for general use but, paradoxically, their introduction has provided a convenient focus for a considerable amount of ill-informed journalistic criticism. E numbers have now been targetted by a number of individuals and self-help groups as a particular cause for concern. While food safety continues to be an important subject, it is also important to maintain a balance between legitimate concerns for safety and the exaggerated assertions of sensationalists. In many cases, an E number has been given to a simple, traditionally used, substance such as acetic acid, lactic acid, caramel, chlorophyll and beetroot red. Others, such as sodium metabisulphite, are not only traditional, but are essential for such common processes as modern wine-making and even the baking of most types of bread. Despite the undisputed fact that occasional reactions can occur to some of these substances, there is no basis for the journalist's use of 'food additive' as a pejorative term or for the allegation that the health of many people is being put at risk by the use of this group of substances.

The boom in the catering industry for 'fast foods' has meant that the use of food additives has increased considerably. For every second of every day, it has been estimated that 200 customers throughout the United States are ordering hamburgers (*Franz, 1987*). The number of fast-food restaurants in the United States rose from 30,000 to 140,000 between 1970 and 1980, and has continued to rise. Fast-food sales of $6.5 billion in 1970 reached a total of $34 billion in 1986, by which time, the worldwide extension of American fast-food chains had invaded Europe, the Far East and the former Soviet Union. In nutritional terms, fast foods have tended to be rich in fat, salt, and calories. This has justifiably caused more concern among nutritionists than the presence of additives.

There has, however, been a marketing response to these areas of public concern. A new trend among fast-food restaurants is to offer salad bars, low-calorie salad dressings, baked potatoes, low-calorie drinks, low-fat hamburgers and low-fat milk. Health education and an emphasis on healthy eating has, thus, had an important influence on public opinion and, by this means, on industrial practice.

Food Ingredients: Fibre

Technical advances in the food-processing industry have been rapid, but an understanding of their implications − both for humans and for livestock − has taken many years to develop. The refining of carbohydrate foods, at first considered to provide substantial advantages, has come to be seen as a mixed blessing. Polished rice was initially regarded as a nutritious product which eliminated the useless husks and made transport easier. It was some years before it was realized that vitamin deficiencies and, in particular, beriberi developed far more readily in Indian populations for whom polished rice had become the staple diet. Refined wheat products, in the form of white flour, appeared to have similar advantages and eliminated the unabsorbable bran residues. Here, also, attitudes have changed and, in this case, the debate has continued since the fifth century BC. There were at least four grades of flour available to the Greeks and Romans, and Hippocrates commented that 'Wholemeal bread cleans out the gut and passes through as excrement. White bread is more nutritious as it makes less faeces' (*Royal College of Physicians, 1980*). The attractiveness and easier baking qualities of white flour, together with the convenient use of bran for animal feeding, continued to commend it to the public at large. There were occasional dissenting voices such as that of Tyron who, in 1683, wrote a book about the value of wholemeal bread as a way to health, long life and happiness. Nevertheless, the popularity of white bread continued through the nineteenth and into most of the present century. Reevaluation has come slowly as the disadvantages of a low-residue diet have come to be appreciated. Gastroenterologists were aware − as Hippocrates had been − that wholemeal bread stimulated bowel activity but, until Burkitt and Trowell (*1975*) stimulated fresh thinking on the subject, white bread, and low-residue diets in general, were considered to play a useful role and to have a therapeutic ability to 'rest the bowel', especially in conditions such as diverticulosis, in which poorly emptying bulges appear between the muscle strips of the bowel wall. Burkitt and Trowell reversed this thinking and suggested that a number of diseases of the West including trends towards constipation, haemorrhoids and varicose veins, were provoked or even caused by low-residue diets. A trend began towards the deliberate reinstatement of unabsorbable fibre as a desirable component of a healthy dietary regime.

It is common to all the various forms of dietary fibre that they are composed mainly of plant cell walls, remain undigested by the gut enzymes, and therefore leave an unabsorbed residue which is the main component of faecal material. Many starches, and stachyose and raffinose from legumes, can also escape absorption in the small bowel and have a laxative effect. Most types of dietary fibre, including wheat bran, are made up of lignin and complex carbohydrates, which are all subject to fermentation and the production of gaseous products. In striking contrast to previous attitudes, it is now widely believed that the removal of these substances is physiologically inept. As the intestine has evolved with a capacity to digest and absorb nutrients and then to discharge unabsorbable food residues, it is proposed that various types of dysfunction can follow if the unabsorbable residues are removed from the food mixture. Seen in this light, a low-residue diet appears to be a paradoxical form of treatment for a condition such as diverticulosis or its associated infected state (diverticulitis). These conditions are seen only in societies that have abandoned the high-fibre type of diet followed in less sophisticated societies. It is now accepted that dietary fibre softens the consistency and increases the volume of the stool, decreases intestinal transit time and alleviates mild constipation. Bran, and dietary fibre in general, is now introduced as a treatment for diverticular disease of the colon in a complete reversal of previous recommendations.

As gastroenterologists accepted Birkett's views and prescribed high-residue diets for their patients with diverticulosis, other claims were made — for example, that pectin and other fibres can lower the serum cholesterol concentration, and help in the management of duodenal ulcer (*Malhotra, 1978*). Studies with pectin and guar gum in the treatment of diabetes mellitus (*Anderson, 1980*) have shown that their presence can modulate the rise in blood glucose levels after glucose loading and stimulate a lower rise in insulin concentration. In diabetics taking guar gum or pectin, reduced therapeutic insulin requirements have been noted. It is now widely accepted that diabetes mellitus is more easily controlled when the patient's diet includes a reasonable content of dietary fibre.

Enthusiasm for fibre reached its peak in the mid-1980s but, despite its importance, its role may have been exaggerated as the pendulum swung too far. Alun Jones and colleagues (*1982*) noted that patients with symptoms of the 'irritable bowel syndrome' sometimes complained that their symptoms became worse when a high-fibre diet was prescribed. It transpired that the intestinal hurry induced by bran may interfere with the absorption of some nutrients, and that the fermentation of unabsorbed food residues in the colon can cause gaseous distention and provoke the problems associated with an irritable bowel, including abdominal pain, colic and distention. It has also been noted (*Macdonald, 1983*) that various types of fibre, including bran, contain phytate, which combines with calcium and other divalent cations to cause deficiencies of these elements in children on a poor diet. Absorption of other nutrients may thus be diminished by bran. The loss of dietary protein which could result may be of significance in underdeveloped countries with populations already on a marginal protein intake.

The 'Saccharine Diseases'

It is by no means a new idea that much of the food eaten in the more developed countries is too refined. In 1966, Cleave published a small book which suggested that refined carbohydrates could have a large number of adverse effects and that abnormally concentrated preparations of these nutrients, together with the loss of other components during the course of food processing, might help to explain the increased incidence of a number of characteristically 'Western' diseases.

Cleave's monograph has undoubtedly stimulated new thinking but, once again, there may have been too great a swing towards the other extreme. Food refinement and processing have now been recognized as the potential cause of a number of problems, but this does not justify the reverse belief that food that has not been processed is more health-giving than the customary mixed Western diet, nor does it suggest that attempts should be made to return to the provision of food which has been grown without the addition of any substances by man.

The terms 'natural', 'organic' and 'health' foods imply a virtue which may not exist, as has been demonstrated when infection has been spread by badly stored preservative-free foods, or when fungus-contaminated peanuts have inadvertently been used. In one study, it was shown that 11 out of 59 samples of 'crunchy' peanut butter from health food producers had over 10 times the recommended maximum content of fungus-derived aflatoxin (*MAFF, 1987*).

Despite the adverse publicity it has received, food processing which has allowed the bulk transport of uncontaminated, uninfected food has undoubtedly been a boon to mankind. Fertilizers, pesticides and the refining processes used in the preparation of food are not only able to make food cheaper, but also more plentiful. Without the use of these substances and of preservatives, it would be difficult or impossible to provide cheap food on a massive scale to underdeveloped countries. Without their use, deficiency diseases and food-borne infections, which still remain a considerable problem in underprivileged communities, may once again achieve uncontrollable proportions.

FOOD AND CORONARY ARTERY DISEASE

Much has still to be learned about the reasons for geographical variations in disease. While the affluent societies are favoured by a relative freedom from malnutrition and the infectious diseases which decimate the childhood populations of underdeveloped communities, those who survive to adult life in impoverished communities are notably free of many of the diseases which predominantly affect Western society. Coronary artery disease is an example of a disorder that has reached epidemic proportions in many developed countries, and our understanding of the dietary factors that contribute to this condition has been slow to progress. The atherosclerotic change in the arteries of the body that underlines this condition is dependent on many factors, and a high intake of saturated fats is a recognized risk factor which appears to have contributed significantly to the rise in prevalence of coronary artery disease. Nevertheless, Eskimos, who have a high fat-intake derived from fish, have a low incidence of coronary artery disorders. The fact that fish oils and fats tend to be unsaturated has therefore led to the suggestion that the avoidance of animal fats, and their replacement with unsaturated fats and fatty acids, may help to prevent the atherosclerotic changes that comprise the main predisposing cause of coronary thrombosis.

A striking fall in the prevalence of coronary artery disease has occurred in the United States as dietary habits have changed and as a trend has developed towards stopping smoking and taking more exercise. In addition, it now appears possible that a diet containing fish may have a protective effect. Lee *et al.* (1985) have shown that fish oils can change the metabolic products of arachidonic acid – for example, from the leukotriene B_4 to the leukotriene B_5 pathway – and that these products of the white blood cells lose much of their inflammatory potential with a diet that is supplemented in this way.

Although a reduction in deaths from coronary artery disease, cancer, and other smoking-related disorders can follow steadily after the introduction of measures to reduce tobacco-smoking in a community, it is clear that dietary and other factors are also important. In line with the evidence produced by Tak Lee, the high fish intake among the Japanese may help to prevent atherosclerotic changes. In contrast, a number of studies have suggested that animal food, and fat in particular, may have an adverse influence. Ironically, recent dietary trends among the Japanese have included a sharp rise in the consumption of animal fat.

When preventive measures are considered, current wisdom suggests a reduction in fat intake, especially saturated fat, and an increase in the intake of vegetables and the more complex carbohydrates, together with an emphasis on increasing physical exercise and a reduction in cigarette-smoking.

Salt and High Blood Pressure

While the Japanese have had a remarkably good health record as far as coronary artery disease is concerned, their susceptibility to the complications of high blood pressure, including stroke, has been notable. Once again, geographical variations in dietary habits may be of importance. A diet which includes salted fish has been proposed as a risk factor and, although there is considerable variation in an individual's ability to handle an excess of sodium in the diet, there is a general agreement that a high salt intake is harmful to hypertensive subjects and that the dietary restriction of salt, or any other form of sodium reduction, may be beneficial. It remains to be seen whether a reduced sodium intake should be regarded as a prophylactic dietary procedure for entire populations, or whether there are at-risk groups which can be identified and given prophylactic dietary advice or asked to reduce their sodium intake early in the development of high blood pressure.

BACK TO NATURE?

There are clearly metabolic differences between individuals that allow one person to consume large quantities of saturated fat with little effect on the serum cholesterol concentration while in another, a smaller intake of fat will cause a great increase in the level of serum cholesterol. The individual's genetic make-up can certainly influence these changes, but genetic effects are also compounded by physiological variables, such as age, gender, and physical and mental activity. There is, however, difficulty in studying the effects of lifestyle, or obtaining evidence of a relationship between nutritional intake and disease, especially because of the long latent period between the development of unhealthy dietary (or other) habits and their undesirable consequences. The high incidence of atheroma in young soldiers killed in Korea suggests an underlying tendency to develop ischaemic heart disease which dates from early life. As noted earlier, however, wartime dietary restrictions can, within a short time, be followed by a fall in the incidence of ischaemic heart disease, only to be followed by a rise when food supplies return to normal. There appears, therefore, to be a case not for a return to nature, but for a return to modest eating habits and an avoidance of the widespread dietary excesses of the affluent West.

While it has been argued that belief in a 'natural' diet is more emotional than logical, it should also be accepted that the tenets of medical orthodoxy should be treated with the same healthy scepticism that was displayed by Cleave and Burkitt. However, a dramatically increased consumption of dietary fibre may be no more healthy than the earlier use of refined foods which almost completely eliminated fibre. The belief that dietary fibre prolongs life is certainly simplistic. As the

16

populations of those countries with a high-fibre intake tend to die at an earlier age than those whose diet contains less fibre, other factors must clearly be taken into account.

A further misconception among those who favour 'natural' diets concerns the value of vitamins. Practitioners of fringe medicine who have used patent preparations containing 'essential' nutrients have long prescribed added vitamins as a form of treatment to supplement natural foods. There is good evidence that the addition of huge doses of vitamins or other essential nutrients ranks with other food fads — their use can be harmful (*Shenkin, 1990*) and cannot be justified.

CONCLUSION

It can be concluded that some of the attention which has focused on food and its dangers has been grossly misdirected and that genuinely adverse reactions to food need to be disentangled from the myths that surround them. On the other hand, the long-term adverse effects of a faulty diet can be serious, and healthy dietary habits need to be more widely promulgated, especially in the developed countries.

Food Intolerance and Attitudes to Food

The farming and gathering of food, and food preparation, serving and eating have a central place in every society in the course of its normal life, its ritual ceremonies, its anxieties and its aspirations. The vital role of food is evident not only when shortages threaten survival, but in the day-to-day life and behaviour of the individual and the family, and in the wider environment of the community. The mother who feeds her child is expressing her love, and the provision of food is a basic aspect of parental care. Food gives gratification and is readily associated with celebration and joy. Over indulgence, on the other hand, carries penalties and, in societies in which women see their shape and weight as an indicator of feminine sexuality, they may restrict and regulate their diet in response to these concepts. This is especially likely to occur in women exposed to the complex social pressures that are a part of Western society.

DEFINITIONS

Because of the central role occupied by food throughout life, a vast number of conditioning factors can affect attitudes to food, both normal and abnormal. These attitudes often condition an individual's perception concerning those foods which are enjoyed, those which are disliked, and those which may cause the unpleasant consequences that are regarded as indicating a 'food reaction'.

If reactions to foods and food additives are to be recognized and distinguished from introspection and incorrect self-diagnosis, they must first be defined. *Food intolerance* (Table 2.1) is a reproducible, unpleasant (adverse) reaction to a specific food or food ingredient that is not psychologically based and occurs even when the food is given in an unidentifiable form. *Food allergy* (Table 2.1) is a form of food intolerance in which there is also evidence of an abnormal immunological reaction to the food – in other words, a reaction similar to that by which the body defends itself against infection or damaging agents.

Other mechanisms can also lead to specific food intolerance. Since the body's digestive processes depend on the enzymes which break down food, intolerance can be caused by a failure of these processes due to enzyme deficiencies (for example, a deficiency of lactase). Causes of food intolerance also include drug-like pharmacological effects (for instance, due to caffeine) as well as toxic effects or those caused by direct irritation (for example, due to gastric acid in the oesophagus). In addition to histamine release, which occurs in the course of an allergic reaction, some foods can lead to the absorption or release of histamine or histamine-like substances by other mechanisms, which are still poorly understood.

The diagnosis of both food intolerance and food allergy relies on the clinical demonstration that a food – even when disguised or encapsulated – causes similar symptoms on repeated occasions. In coeliac disease (see Chapter 9), which is characterized by an intolerance to the gluten component of wheat and other cereal grains, another test

Table 2.1 Food intolerance and food allergy

	Allergy	Intolerance (other than allergy)	Food aversion (or avoidance)
Open challenge	+	+	±
Blinded challenge	+	+	−
Immunological abnormality	+	−	−

+ = positive result; − = negative result; ± = variable result.

may be substituted. Microscopic examination of the lining of the small bowel — as sampled through a swallowed endoscope — shows a flattening of the filaments (villi) which is usually assumed to be the result of the gluten sensitivity unless proved otherwise.

Food aversion comprises both psychological food avoidance — when the subject has psychological motives for avoiding a particular food — and psychological intolerance, which is an unpleasant bodily reaction caused by emotions associated with the food rather than the food itself. In such a case, the symptoms occur consistently when the food is recognized, but not when given in an unrecognizable form. The symptoms may be indirectly provoked, for example, when an apprehensive patient overbreathes and loses excessive amounts of carbon dioxide during expiration, thus inducing an alkalosis. In this case, giddiness, a rapid pulse, nausea, weakness, tingling of the hands and feet, and thought disturbances may be the chief complaints. These are symptoms of the *hyperventilation syndrome*.

EPIDEMIOLOGY

The distribution of food intolerance in the population at large may be extremely difficult to assess because of a lack of practical diagnostic methods applicable within a population survey. The use of question-naires may identify self-diagnosed people who believe they are affected, but this cannot be of real value unless the errors of self-diagnosis are assessed. The symptoms which can be produced by foods and food additives vary, and the 'gold standard' for diagnosis is the controlled challenge test in which, at different times, the suspected food and another substance indistinguishable from it are given to the patient, and the consequences observed. To prevent the food being recognized, it may be necessary to encapsulate it or arrange tube-feeding. Diagnostic methods are therefore cumbersome, and tests to establish their validity cannot easily be carried out on the scale needed for a population study. Lacking this diagnostic information, most epidemi-ologists are obliged to use unreliable diagnostic data, and the conclusions that can be drawn are limited.

The replies that have been gathered from questionnaires suggest that 4.5% to 33% of the population regard themselves as being prone to food allergy or intolerant reactions. When further proof is sought through challenge tests and close observation after taking the food in question, much lower figures are obtained. The frequency of food reactions after challenge tests appears to be of the order of 1.4–1.9% (*Young, 1992*). By the same criteria, food additive intolerance is around 10 times less common (*Young et al., 1987*).

More precise figures have emerged in the few conditions in which the diagnosis is more soundly based. Gluten intolerance due to coeliac disease is usually severe enough to require hospital investigation, and the finding of flattened villi in the small bowel is virtually diagnostic. Lactose intolerance is another condition for which there is a simple diagnostic method, the breath hydrogen test. In this case, a dose of lactose is swallowed and, provided that it is not digested, it is eventually fermented in the large bowel to produce gases which include hydrogen. This hydrogen is then absorbed and released in the breath, where it can be measured. The frequency of lactose intolerance in adult Caucasian populations is 5%, but higher figures (50–80%) have been reported in some African and Asian communities. Other intolerant reactions – for example, to biogenic amines – are now being identified, but there is no reliable estimate of their frequency.

A recent study of the population of High Wycombe has shown a marked contrast between the public's perception of food-induced reactions and their prevalence as demonstrated by specific testing. Questionnaires were sent (*Young et al., 1987*) to one in 10 of the people on a local electoral register, and replies were received from 18,582 people, representing 62% of those canvassed. Of those who replied, 2890 (15.6%) considered that they had an unpleasant reaction caused by specific foods; 1372 (7.4%) thought they reacted to food additives, and most (1074) of these subjects believed that they reacted to specific foods as well as food additives.

The study then focused on the food additive problem. Individual claims were cross-checked by interviews, clinical assessment and, where appropriate, a series of daily challenge tests, in which capsules of either food additives or inert (placebo) substances were given over a 20-day period. As neither the patient nor the doctor was aware of the contents of the capsules taken, the trial was 'double-blind'. As both the test substances and inert placebos were taken in the capsules, the trial was 'placebo-controlled'. At the end of this trial, only three individuals were observed to have an adverse reaction to the additives used. Although these data have yet to be supplemented by the results of further challenge tests with sodium metabisulphite and monosodium glutamate, this was a clear indication that many of those who believed they experienced reactions to food additives were basing their comments on a misconception. The final estimate of the prevalence of food additive intolerance in this population was between 0.01–0.23%, which corresponds well with other available figures.

EATING HABITS

There is a wide variation in food intake and energy expenditure not only between individuals, but also in the same individual at different times. This is particularly true of adolescents, possibly because of their rapid growth at that age, but also, in part, because of the effects of immature emotions on appetite.

A study of the eating habits of 16- and 17-year-old schoolgirls (*Lacey et al., 1978*) showed that there was a marked variation in food intake, especially of carbohydrates, and that disorders of eating behaviour were widespread. Food intake tended to increase prior to menstruation and to fall immediately after it, mainly because of changes in carbohydrate intake, while the ingestion of protein and fat remained more stable. In addition, there were marked variations from one day to the next, with a tendency for the girls to eat up to four times as much on particular days, especially during the weekend. Most girls had episodes in which carbohydrate intake was low followed by a period of increased eating, mainly of carbohydrate foods. In some, the pattern was more dramatic and could be regarded as 'binge eating'. This pattern is now known as bulimia (*Crisp, 1981*). In addition, up to 5% of women induce vomiting periodically as a means of controlling body weight (*Lacey, 1983*).

The distinction between food faddism, bulimia and 'dieting' may be difficult to make and, in their milder forms, dieting – and even bulimia – are almost universal in young women in Western societies. Fashionable concepts of body shape in these cultures have so conditioned their attitudes that the majority of women try to conform to the ideal female shape which, since World War II, has become more angular and lean. The notional shape of a woman has, however, fluctuated through the ages. Lacey has noted that the shape of Hollywood actresses in the 1930s differed markedly from that of Twiggy, a fashion model of the 1960s, or from the shape of women in other cultures who, to be attractive, must show the rounded figure that is associated with prosperity and success. Within a given community, there may also be an excessive pressure to slim among specific groups of women – for example, ballet dancers and fashion models – which appears to make them more susceptible to dieting, faddism and bulimia. A few patients are male and some jockeys – under pressure to remain thin – have been reported to develop bulimic symptoms which vary with the season and the sporting calendar (*King & Mezey*, 1987).

There is a fine shading between attempts to control body weight and an attitude towards those foods which are acceptable and those which are not, or those which are perceived as unhealthy or the cause of harmful reactions in the body. Food fads are particularly common in the infant, the adolescent, and in those under stress. The concern of a parent to feed a child well may conflict with the infant's urge to assert an increasing autonomy. Acceptance and rejection of food in infancy are the earliest expressions of the child's will, and particular foods may come to be singled out as tokens of comfort or offence.

When a particular food becomes invested with emotion, a fad or craving for that food can lead to a pathological response in which the reaction to sadness or discomfort is acted upon by the passive response of eating. Childhood obesity may then become not a sign of good mothering, but a reflection of a mother's anxieties. As the child grows older, the search for foods which are, for example, sweet, or which provide a sense of fullness, can reinforce the symbolic attitudes to food learned in infancy. Current nostrums, especially concerning allergic causes of ill health, encourage these neurotic attitudes.

In recent years, the pronouncements of a few misguided medical advisers has led, in several cases, to the progression of faddism and the rejection of an ever-widening range of foods on the grounds that they are the cause of a 'total allergy' syndrome. The rejection of foods, sometimes reinforced by parental preoccupations, shows some similarities to the induced starvation seen in anorexia nervosa. In contrast to the latter condition, however, an abnormal concern about body shape and anxieties about the developing features of adolescence appear to play no part.

THE EATING DISORDERS

Massive obesity, bulimia, and anorexia nervosa all involve mental attitudes in which the patient displaces her (or, occasionally, his) emotions onto food and the effects which it may have on the body. The fact that women are predominantly affected emphasizes the relationship to sexuality. A healthy woman has twice as much body fat as a man; the first rapid increase in fat deposition occurs at puberty. A man has one-and-a-half times the lean body mass and one-and-a-half times the bone mass of a woman (*Brook, 1981*). As the girl at puberty develops her first sexual emotions together with a dramatic change in shape and weight, and the onset of menstruation, this preparation for adult womanhood and reproductive capacity changes her relationships to others and can exacerbate feelings of stress and insecurity.

The concept of the desirable female shape still differs in different parts of the world. The voluptuous rounded forms depicted by Rubens are still fashionable in many societies where the Western doctor who advocates a healthy reducing diet is listened to with polite scepticism.

In a study of Swedish teenagers who were asked if they thought themselves too fat, 25% of the 14-year-olds and over 50% of the 18-year-olds regarded themselves as fat. Only 7% of 18-year-old boys put themselves into this category (*Nylander, 1971*). Three-quarters of the older groups had made serious efforts to diet, although only small losses of body weight were reported. Nevertheless, a number of symptoms may have been associated with this deliberate dietary manipulation, including amenorrhoea. In addition, food fads, dietary manipulation or compulsive overeating were frequently accompanied by an increased interest in food and food preparation.

Food Faddism

Abnormal attitudes to food can develop at any age. Food refusal in infancy is often part of a more general rejection or negative response. The battle of wills between parent and infant can lead to later problems as parents become anxious about proper feeding and the infant becomes aware of its own urge to independence (*Berry Brazelton, 1976*). As an infant focuses on the refusal of certain foods or reverts to demanding to be fed by his mother or by a bottle, the conflict may be heightened.

When food is an expression of a mother's love for her child, attempts to reject that food – or to insist upon its delivery – can induce emotional overtones of a high order.

The development of these trends in later childhood can give emotional values to selected foods, or may be used by the mother to console and comfort a distressed child. When sweet or starchy foods are used in this way, the 'fad' can become a persisting, abnormal feature of the intimate relationship between mother and child. When food is provided as a response to sadness or discomfort, childhood obesity may then be a reflection of the mother's anxiety or insecurity. Lacey (1983) has pointed out that, as the child gets older, the manifestation of a neurotic faddism can range from a whim to a freakish craze.

It is a small step from fads of this kind to the concept of allergic reactions, either real or imagined. Under the fashionable pressures of journalistic enthusiasm, the search for a food culprit on which to blame a child's symptoms may take on an obsessional dimension. The pursuit of this type of faddism can lead to the exclusion of either a single food or a wide range of foods to the point where the complications of malnutrition may appear, including vitamin deficiencies or frank scurvy (*Hughes et al., 1986*).

Anorexia, Bulimia and Obesity

Anorexia nervosa is an eating disorder in which food is refused, if necessary by subterfuge. Other turbulent eating patterns, as noted above, include the bulimic syndrome, in which there may be both food binges and an accompanying tendency to induce vomiting to correct feelings of bloating or of guilt. Abnormal attitudes to food are also found in grossly obese people who, for the most part, overeat at times of emotional distress, but otherwise tend to have fewer meals with a lower calorie content than people of normal weight (*Hawkins, 1979*).

The relationship between fat and female sexuality has been emphasized by the fat deposition which occurs not only in the pubescent girl, but also during pregnancy and sometimes at the menopause. The biological function of fat as a storage tissue can provide a reserve of nutrients during pregnancy and lactation which may, however, be jeopardized at times of fat depletion. The endocrine changes which follow food deprivation can suppress menstruation and ovulation, thereby diminishing the risk of pregnancy in an individual whose fat stores may be seriously depleted. These changes serve as a biological protection against further depletion of the energy stores and, by delaying puberty or suppressing ovarian function, prevent the metabolic demands of child-bearing. The pubescent girl who develops anorexia nervosa may have become aware that dieting can suppress the expressions of sexuality of which she is afraid.

Anorexia nervosa

The word 'anorexia' means a lack of appetite, but the main concern of the anorectic is a morbid fear of becoming fat and a determination, therefore, to maintain a low body weight. The motivation which leads to this fear is complex; she may be experiencing the emotional turmoil associated with her first sexual emotions, the dramatic change in her weight and shape, the commencement of menstruation, and the changing relationships which begin to develop both inside and outside her family. What may begin as a tentative refusal of food may progress to other measures, which can include self-induced vomiting, purgation or excessive exercise to maintain a weight loss of 25% or more of the original body weight. It is characteristic that menstrual periods may cease (and perhaps a loss of libido in the few men who develop this condition). The pulse rate slows, a fine growth of short lanugo hair develops over the body, and the anorectic is characteristically very alert, bright-eyed and even frenetically active. In the current climate in which 'food allergy' has become a fashionable diagnosis, claims may also be made about illness patterns being provoked by particular foods.

As a variation of the anorectic theme, there are a few patients who are both bulimic and anorectic. These subjects often show marked swings of body weight. As the weight rises above a threshold of around 43 kg, the bulimic anorectic may confess to redeveloping sexual feelings of which she is terrified. Carbohydrate avoidance and other features of anorectic behaviour may then supervene in a patient who, in most cases, is likely to show other evidence of being very disturbed.

Bulimia

For the mature woman, the preparation of food and the need to feed her family may play a central role in her life. Food, which may be offered as a token of comfort and love to her young, may also come to be seen as an available source of comfort to herself at times of stress. Whether for this or other reasons, bingeing with food can, in some women, appear to provide the relief of tension which men are more likely to seek through binges of alcohol. Nevertheless, most bulimics have either a normal or a near-normal body weight. It is not uncommon for foods to be avoided for some time, only to be seized upon in a gluttonous binge on a later occasion. Periods of weight gain are then controlled by further dieting, laxative abuse, or self-induced vomiting.

The bulimic patient who binges characteristically hides in a particular room, and other members of the family may never suspect the indulgences which occur behind closed doors. Before a bulimic episode, the patient may have a feeling of excitement associated with a craving which is eventually satisfied by the bingeing episode. This is followed by a feeling of bloating, guilt and humiliation, which may be relieved by vomiting. This usually provides a sense of reassurance as it is seen as an effective means of preventing weight gain, sometimes after dieting attempts, laxatives, diuretics or slimming pills have failed. When laxatives or diuretics are used, a depletion of potassium and sodium may cause problems. Menstrual irregularities are very common.

Bulimic episodes are sometimes a reaction to episodes of emotional stress or domestic conflict. The addition of induced vomiting, however, has been proposed by Lacey (*1983*) as a middle-class phenomenon to prevent the development of what otherwise may become a progressive and massive obesity.

Massive obesity
The development of massive obesity is even more complex. It is commonly associated with sexual inactivity and often has implications for the marital relationship. Lacey has noted that most massively obese women marry when they are already grossly overweight, so that marriage is embarked upon with awareness of all of the implications that massive obesity has.

Characteristically, the trend towards obesity begins in infancy and childhood. The relationship itself between the obese child and the mother is unusual, as a mother with both normal and obese children may persist in giving excessively large meals to her clearly overweight child while ignoring medical advice. The emotional background of such a relationship is characteristically very ambivalent.

In adults, moderate obesity is not associated with psychological disturbances. Indeed, there is some evidence (*Crisp & McGuinness,*

1976) that people who are up to about 50% above their ideal weight are less emotionally disturbed than those of average weight and certainly than those who are thin. It does not follow that patients who are sufficiently concerned about themselves to attend obesity clinics are in this category. As individuals who have decided to conquer their obesity, they are more likely to indulge in prolonged dietary restriction which may, in itself, lead to changes in mood, particularly to depression.

The role of massive obesity in depressing sexual activity is notable. Obese women can sometimes pinpoint the onset of a rapidly progressive obesity to a time of sexual molestation, notably at the time of puberty. There is, however, difficulty in disentangling the many factors that may contribute to problems of this kind.

Psychiatric Illness and Food

The relationship between psychological problems and attitudes to food has been well delineated. It is sometimes claimed, however, that much psychiatric ill health and depression are induced by food allergy and can be relieved by diet (see Chapter 3). While many of the claims that have been made do not stand up to critical examination, mood changes are common in patients with coeliac disease, both treated and untreated. While the need for rigid adherence to a sometimes distasteful diet may be a distressing feature of this disease, and untreated patients may be moody because they feel unwell, this may not be the whole story. Schizophrenia has been claimed to be more common among coeliac patients, possibly in connection to the impaired metabolism of tyrosine or because of a toxic effect of the peptides derived from gluten (see Chapter 9). In addition, irritability and bad behaviour in milk-allergic children can sometimes disappear with dietary treatment, together with the asthma, eczema and other manifestations which are the clinical hallmarks of the allergy (*Buisseret, 1978*).

If it is accepted that mental changes can accompany gluten enteropathy, and that a change in behaviour can follow the treatment of food allergy in a child, it is appropriate that the possible effects of food allergy in provoking psychiatric ill health in adults should be put to the test. Rix and his colleagues (*1984*) carried out a psychiatric study of 23 adult patients who believed that they were suffering from food allergy (excluding cases of urticaria). What Rix *et al.* found was that 19 of these subjects had psychological causes for their illness, but no evidence of organic food hypersensitivity whatsoever. There was also a strikingly high prevalence of common neurotic symptoms in these patients. The remaining four individuals had proven food-related skin reactions or asthma. As measured by a psychiatric symptom-scoring system (*Goldberg et al., 1970*), these four individuals had no evidence of psychiatric disorder or food-related psychological symptoms.

While children may respond differently (see below), a sound case for accepting food allergy as a cause of psychiatric illness in adults has yet to be established, and individual cases in which this claim is made should be carefully examined. In patients who present with overt psychiatric symptoms, food fads or obsessional neuroses concerning food, it is therefore imperative to apply formal diagnostic criteria and to seek evidence of associated allergic manifestations or immunological abnormalities before accepting a self-diagnosis of food allergy.

Childhood Hyperactivity: Food-Related or Yet Another 'Attitude'?

Much publicity has been given to the concept that 'food allergy' is responsible for a wide range of otherwise unexplainable symptoms. It has been claimed, in particular, that colouring agents used in foods – or the foods themselves – can cause childhood behaviour disorders, thus justifying the concept of 'childhood hyperactivity'. As a fashionable label, this diagnosis is on the wane, but the basis for it needs to be examined. Hyperactivity may be loosely defined as a condition associated with constant restlessness, disorganization and inattention but, as agreed-upon norms for activity levels and attention are lacking, there is some doubt as to whether hyperactivity is a discrete condition or simply a collection of non-specific behaviour problems common to many psychiatric disorders, especially in childhood. Speculative explanations which have been put forward include the suggestion that zinc or vitamin deficiencies might be the cause; that an abnormal response to sugar or yeast is involved (*Bock, 1986*); that some cases are due to brain damage or malfunction; or that food colours may be responsible. While parents are sometimes pleased to be told that there is a physical cause for their child's problem, most double-blind studies with food additives have produced either totally negative results (*Mattes & Gittelman, 1981*) or mostly negative results, while suggesting that a few younger children may do better with a restricted diet (*Harley et al.,* *1978a; 1978b*). In a further study which tested a different hypothesis, childhood behaviour disorders which had been attributed to 'sugar reactions' were not confirmed when a challenge dose of sugar was given blind (*Rapoport, 1982–3*).

Some of the confusion which surrounds this issue stems from the fact that children who are diagnosed as hyperactive in some countries are most likely to be labelled as having a conduct disorder in others. Estimates of the numbers affected also vary; the figures derived from teacher questionnaire surveys suggest that 5–20% of inner-city children may be affected, whereas figures derived from the clinical diagnoses made upon children attending psychiatric clinics suggest that 0.1% of this population are affected. Complaints of a child's hyperactive behaviour are common reasons for referral to a child psychiatrist, especially in boys, who are referred four times more frequently than girls.

Although there are differences of terminology used by child psychiatrists in North America and in the United Kingdom, 'overactivity' generally implies an excess of physical activity which is, nevertheless, within the boundaries of normal. 'Hyperactivity' or 'attention-deficit disorder with hyperactivity' consists of excessive activity, a lack of attention and impulsiveness. The 'hyperkinetic syndrome' refers to symptoms of sufficient severity to lead to developmental delay, usually commencing before 6 years of age in the absence of other inborn or acquired disease.

It is interesting to consider how the food link came to be established in the absence of solid evidence. Most of the work that has been carried out dates from Feingold's (1975) hypothesis that food additives and naturally occurring salicylate are the causes of hyperactivity. Although unsupported by sound data, this led to widespread publicity and uncritical public acceptance which has resulted in the formation of numerous support groups advocating elimination diets for hyperactive children. It is a matter of concern that, for example, the recommended remedial diets do not contain the low levels of salicylate intended, but this and other criticisms may not deter the supporters of this approach. A view quoted by Rippere (1983) is that 'The biggest danger to the Feingold approach . . . is that it so frequently doesn't work and that its failures can lead parents to give up the search for something in the environment that is producing the problem behaviour.'

Claims concerning the effects of food on mental processes cannot, however, be dismissed without further examination. Apart from the occasional association of coeliac disease with mental illness and the association of food allergy with irritable behaviour, it cannot be denied that alertness and mental function can be influenced by dietary factors. Potentially toxic doses of caffeine (above 250 mg) can easily be ingested in every-day life, where a cup of coffee may contain 100 mg of caffeine and a cup of tea 60 mg. Children, who are more sensitive to these effects, can obtain up to 60 mg of caffeine in cola drinks.

In adults, moderate doses of caffeine stimulate mental activity and reduce fatigue, but can also provoke nervousness, irritability, agitation, tremulousness and headache. Heavy coffee drinkers may complain of poor sleep at night, cardiac arrhythmias, nausea, vomiting and, because of its diuretic effect, a change in bowel habit, with constipated stools, abdominal pain and sometimes diarrhoea. Caffeine withdrawal symptoms of irritability, nervousness, nausea and a further exacerbation of headache have also been described.

Other associations between food reactions and mental changes have been noted. Intolerance to food proteins can cause mental confusion or affect intellectual function in children with inborn metabolic diseases, such as phenylketonuria. While most of these conditions are rare, when they do occur, malaise, restlessness and irritability can follow the ingestion of food. The possibility that behavioural problems can be caused by food or food-additive intolerance should therefore not be dismissed without proper consideration of the evidence on an individual basis.

Because of the continuing controversy and widespread public concern over these claims, some of the most publicized work deserves further analysis – despite the many carefully conducted studies which have given negative results. A complex study at the Great Ormond Street Hospital in London (*Egger et al., 1985*) claimed to have observed a dramatic effect on the hyperactive behaviour of a very unusual group of children, including many who also had eczema, asthma and epilepsy. Those who improved on a restricted diet were given various foods and food additives, including tartrazine in a large dose of 150 mg daily for 1 week. Although no child reacted to tartrazine alone, 27 deteriorated during the 1-week challenge period and eight of these did so in subsequent double-blind challenge tests. Most patients reacted to several foods, and 46 other provocative agents were identified.

These findings differed remarkably from other published studies, and there were also large unexplained differences depending on the order in which the challenge tests were given. A more recently published paper on this controversial topic (*Pollock & Warner, 1990*) has reviewed the extensive and largely negative literature. The authors' own contribution included a challenge study involving 39 children whose parents reported that noticeable behaviour changes followed deliberate or accidental food-additive ingestion, usually within 2 hours or so. Capsules of similar appearance were then given to the children every morning for 7 weeks. For 2 weeks of the 7, the capsules contained 125 mg of four azo colours (active preparations); during the remaining 5 weeks, the capsules contained lactose (placebo). Behaviour scores were recorded by parents and showed very little change in the average behaviour score during the challenge which, however, most parents were unable to detect. There were no effects on the more general symptoms, such as wheezing, rash or other physical changes, and there was no association with allergy. It therefore appeared to be possible that there was a minimal effect on the behaviour of a small minority of hyperactive children but, in general, this was of dubious relevance. At the very least, parents who believed that their children were hyperactive because of an effect of food additives were nearly always mistaken, a view which was strongly endorsed by Rowe (*1988*) after a review of the Australian literature and 220 personal cases. Nevertheless, Rowe found two children – both with other allergic features – who became irritable and developed sleep disturbances when given artificial colours. One child who appeared to have a sustained, partial improvement on a restricted diet still continued to have some behavioural disorders, and had a long history of learning difficulties and easily provoked aggression.

In a further study of 19 children with a definitive history of respiratory, dermatological or behavioural symptoms induced by artificial yellow food-colouring, Wilson and Scott (*1989*) could find none who developed changes of behaviour after drinks which contained the colours, although one developed urticaria and migraine, and another asthma and abdominal pain. Unexpectedly, one child developed behavioural disturbances after taking preservatives.

While there may still be room for doubt in exceptional cases, the studies carried out by David (1987, 1988) have summarized an impression for which much evidence has now accumulated. In general, the avoidance of additives has not been shown to have more than a short-lived effect on behaviour, although irritability, restlessness, and a loss of concentration is not uncommon in children who have asthma or eczema and are subject to sleep disturbances.

In view of the intensive regimens which have been recommended on the basis of so many incorrect diagnoses, some principles of management should be emphasized. It is important that children should not be given elimination diets without a good indication. The continuation of an inappropriate diet by way of treatment is socially restricting; indeed, diets may be employed as a form of punishment. When restricted diets are used, nutritional inadequacies can arise and there is the need for supervision by a dietitian. More important, since hyperactive behaviour can have many causes, the use of an inappropriate diet may lead to the neglect of psychosocial and other factors.

A common criticism of conventional medicine is that insufficient time is available for consultation and a detailed assessment of the child's environment and developmental history, which may form an important part of the therapeutic process. When behavioural problems are severe or associated with learning problems, an explanation to the parents may not be enough. The child may require assessment by a clinical psychologist or a psychiatrist and psychological or sometimes pharmacological treatment. If parents have already tried diet and believe it has helped, it should be relaxed after a period to see if symptoms return as, in the few cases of food-additive intolerance in association with urticaria, the intolerance has nearly always proved to be transient (Pollock & Warner, 1987).

Blinded food-additive challenges are helpful, particularly in convincing parents that a diet is unnecessary but, if parents insist on food-additive elimination, behaviour should be documented before and during the diet, after which blinded food-additive challenges should be made. A misleading impression may be due not only to the placebo effect of such trials, but also to the extra attention that a child receives during a dietary regime which can, in itself, be beneficial, although counterbalanced by the many adverse effects of elimination diets. The main methods of treatment for hyperactivity are still psychological, reinforced if necessary by the use of drug therapy. A false emphasis upon diet can be comforting to the parents, but harmful to the child.

CONCLUSION

The confusion which has arisen in the study of food reactions begins with the many different — and false — interpretations which have been put upon words such as 'allergy'. While food allergy does exist, and should be clearly defined and recognized, this diagnosis should not be used to prevent the recognition of emotional overtones which, from infancy onwards, have made food the frequent object of anxiety, emotion and conflict. Food faddism, childhood behavioural problems, faulty eating habits and the metabolic effects of hyperventilation may all, on occasions, be misinterpreted as an adverse response to food or food additives. Attitudes to body shape may add to the problem, especially in those who fear obesity or in girls who are anxious about the changes in body shape associated with their emerging sexuality.

If further confusion is to be prevented, there is a need to acknowledge the wide range of other possible causes in people who claim to have food-induced symptoms and to recognize the various ways in which these different conditions can be presented.

CHAPTER
—3—

Food and Alternative Medicine

ECOLOGY AND THE PROTEST MOVEMENT

Concerned with the damage to the environment produced by man and by modern living, the ecology movement and its heirs, the political Green Parties of Europe and the United States, have focused on the environmental issues which have been of increasing concern to large numbers of people. The medical offshoot of the ecology movement has a more chequered history. When clinical ecologists emphasized the dangers that may arise from pollutants in our atmosphere, and in our drinking water and food, their concerns were similar to those of the medical profession in general, and of the specialities of public health medicine and occupational medicine in particular. The clinical ecology movement has now gone much further and has made assertions concerning environmental disease which are not based on objective evidence, but have, in fact, become articles of faith. It is at this point that conventional medicine and clinical ecology part company.

The concept of 'environmental illness' or 'chemical hypersensitivity syndrome' (*Magarian, 1982*) is based on the assumption that environmental chemicals and foods are responsible for a type of illness which can present in an unlimited variety of ways in the absence of objective physical changes or abnormal laboratory tests. As the journal *Clinical Ecology* states in each of its issues, 'Ecological illness is a polysymptomatic, multisystem chronic disorder manifested by adverse reactions to environmental excitants, as they are modified by individual susceptibility in terms of specific adaptations.' In claiming a particular skill in dealing with medical problems associated with environmental damage, clinical ecologists have attracted a sympathetic press, especially when they have stated that they can diagnose and treat conditions which defeat their more conventional medical colleagues. It may, therefore, be appropriate to analyse the problems of pollution and environmental damage in more detail before considering whether the views of ecologists and other practitioners of alternative medicine should be taken more seriously.

The Problems of Pollution

It is now widely accepted that there is a need for more rigorous control of atmospheric pollution. Indeed, the more general problems of pollution have been of increasingly widespread concern from the time, in 1956, when 35 deaths occurred from industrial mercurial contamination of the fish in Minimata Bay (*Rafflle et al., 1987*). In campaigning for better standards to prevent the contamination of food, public health physicians and industrial medicine specialists have also given a lead which has been widely followed and has helped to prevent the transmission of infection by food, water and milk. By encouraging food testing, they have also helped to track down and prevent some of the scandals of recent years, such as the deliberate addition of ethylene glycol (antifreeze) to Austrian wine or the addition of potentially toxic amounts of wood alcohol or methylisothiocyanate to cheap wines from Italy (*Skipworth, 1992*). The key to the success of these efforts has depended on better hygiene, better methods of storage, the monitoring of contaminants in food and drink, and the establishment of safe methods for the preservation of food.

It is at this point that clinical ecologists have taken issue with their colleagues by suggesting that the very methods which help food storage and make food more widely available carry considerable dangers of their own. While avoiding scientific studies which could help to establish the presence or absence of harmful substances, the more enthusiastic clinical ecologists have pressed for a virtual ban on the use of food additives – whether as preservatives or for any other purpose – and have distracted attention from other problems which need to be addressed. A number of clinical procedures have also been invented which claim to 'desensitize' the victims of environmental damage to the foods and other environmental agents which have caused their problems. Basic to this approach is the assumption that the body's oversensitive, 'allergic' reaction is the cause of the problem and that an immunological deficiency is involved. No useful evidence has been produced to support these contentious explanations or to justify the prescription of costly and unproven remedial treatments over long periods of time.

Much of the atmospheric pollution that has occurred in industrial areas has aroused concern because of substances which are either irritants or toxic. Oxides of nitrogen and volatile organic compounds from car exhaust fumes can lead to photochemical pollution by reacting, in the presence of sunlight, to produce ozone. Low ozone levels, similar to those occurring in urban areas, have now been shown to potentiate the tendency of allergic asthmatic subjects to react to ragweed or grass pollen (*Molfino et al., 1991*). Sulphur dioxide, ozone, and car exhaust fumes in the environments of Los Angeles, Tokyo or Syracuse have often proved intolerable to healthy people, and the effects of atmospheric pollution have been especially dramatic in the region of the burning oil wells of Kuwait where, in 1991, it was sometimes difficult to distinguish night from day.

Atmospheric pollution is particularly intolerable to patients with preexisting lung disease or asthma, and it is notable that such diseases are becoming more common. In the United Kingdom in 1946, asthma was diagnosed in 6.2 per 1000 firstborn between the ages of 0–4 years. In a follow-up study of this 1946 cohort of children, their firstborn offspring were diagnosed as having asthma three times more frequently (*Wadsworth, 1985*). Independent evidence of the increased importance of asthma is seen in the recorded mortality rate for asthma in England and Wales which has risen by an average annual rate of 4.7% over the years 1974–1984, most strikingly in the group aged 5–34 years. This increase cannot be explained by changes in diagnostic practice, and similar increases have been reported in Melbourne, where a 1964 survey has been repeated after an interval of 26 years (*Robertson et al., 1991*).

While there is still little evidence of any serious health hazards caused by modern agricultural methods or food processing, there has been a growing concern over environmental pollution in the United Kingdom. In response to this concern, the Department of the

Environment has set up an 'Air Quality Helpline' through which it is possible to obtain information on levels of pollutants in the United Kingdom (*Acheson, 1991*).

Asthma and eczema (*Taylor et al., 1984*) stand out as very striking examples of conditions which, against the trend of virtually all other treatable disorders, have become more common. Direct toxic effects on the bronchial mucosa are clearly contributory, but there is now good evidence that the effects of bronchial irritants and of allergy can potentiate one another (*Molfino et al., 1991*). Direct toxic effects can explain some cases but, in others, there appears to be an allergic response to a food or environmental agent. The mechanism responsible for the asthma can vary but, apart from the causes mentioned, the British Industrial Injuries Advisory Council now recognizes seven groups of substances which can cause occupational asthma: platinum salts, isocyanates, epoxy resins, colophony fumes, proteolytic enzymes, laboratory animals, and grain (or flour) dust. A number of highly reactive industrial chemicals can thus cause asthma either by their toxicity or by provoking an allergic reaction, or by a combination of both (*Newman Taylor, 1987*). The list has now been extended to include any sensitizing agent inhaled at work, including pharmaceutical products, wood dust and castor bean dust (*Burge, 1990*). It cannot be assumed that a particular substance will always cause the same type of adverse reaction.

Historically speaking, the respiratory effects of industrial smog and of the old-fashioned 'pea-soup' fog of English cities were too obvious to be ignored. Modern pollutants are usually less visible, but the transformation of Japan into an industrial superpower has highlighted the damage which can be caused, and has led the courts in Osaka to award over a billion pounds in damages to the victims of air pollution (*Popham, 1991*). While there may also be more insidious effects of lower levels of pollution, these remain to be assessed. What evidence there is suggests that traffic fumes, industrial and domestic pollutants, ventilation plants, tobacco smoke, ozone, natural allergens and food additives all help, to some extent, to provoke bronchial hyperreactivity or potentiate allergic reactions, thereby providing a basis for the development of asthma and other adverse effects. There is increasing evidence that this is not only a problem of the West, but also of those Third World countries which acquire Western habits (*Turner, 1987*).

The difficulty in analysing the mechanisms that cause clinical reactions is especially apparent in reactions provoked by food. As sulphur dioxide can provoke asthma when inhaled (*Harries et al., 1981*), it has been assumed that a direct irritant effect is responsible when food-induced asthma is provoked by foods which contain either free sulphur dioxide or sodium metabisulphite as a preservative (*Baker et al., 1981*). There is some evidence, however, that sulphites can also trigger an allergic response (*Wolf & Nicklas, 1985*). Whatever the mechanism, a food additive can be firmly implicated, and it must be accepted that some asthmatics need to avoid food, wine or other drinks which contain this preservative. Cow's milk and other natural, unprocessed foods can also provoke asthmatic attacks (*Lessof et al., 1980; Papageorgiou et al., 1983*) and, in fact, adverse reactions to natural foods are far more common than those to metabisulphite or other food additives (*Young et al., 1987*). Just as no single mechanism can explain all the illnesses provoked by food or environmental agents, so no single group of substances can be considered to be predominantly at fault.

FOOD AND THE COUNTERREVOLUTION

Much of the evidence quoted above has been fully accepted by chest physicians, immunologists and allergists. There have been well documented instances where grossly contaminated food has resulted in illness or death on an epidemic scale, and many less severe outbreaks in which contaminated food has been suspected, but never proved. The industrial contamination of the water in Minamata Bay took much investigational effort before the cause of the disaster was identified. The contamination of cooking oil has also caused outbreaks of poisoning due to tricresyl phosphate, and these were no easier to track down. When small amounts of methylenedianiline penetrated into some sacks of flour that were being transported in a van at Epping, only the most diligent research identified the cause of the 84 cases of jaundice which followed (*Raffle et al., 1987*). The same applied to an outbreak of acute gastroenteritis in Vermont which led to the realization that heavy metals can cause problems, as when acidic foods are stored in copper, tin or galvanized containers (*Centers for Disease Control, 1977*).

Toxic effects can also be combined with the indirect consequences of the body's hypersensitive reactions. When contaminated rapeseed oil was responsible for an outbreak of 'toxic-allergic' syndrome (*Tabuenca, 1981*), symptoms as varied as fever, rash, muscle pain, headache and drowsiness were seen in combination with evidence of interstitial pneumonitis, lymphadenopathy, hepatosplenomegaly, cerebral oedema, eosinophilia, and a rise in serum aldolase (*Kilbourne et al., 1983*). The increase in circulating white blood cells, identifiable by eosin staining (eosinophilia), suggested that an allergic reaction might be involved and, as a further indicator of an allergic response, 43% had a raised serum immunoglobulin E (IgE) level (see Chapter 5). Many continued to develop a chronic illness, possibly caused by the release of toxic oleoanilides from damaged cells.

This 'toxic-oil syndrome' showed some remarkable similarities to the symptoms seen in patients in the United States in 1989 who, after being given products containing L-tryptophan, developed a chronic illness in which eosinophilia and muscle pains (myalgia) were the most prominent features (*Kaufman et al., 1991*). It appeared, however, that exposure to the provoking agent was not the only factor and that the genetic make-up of the individual might play a part. The same applied to those who consumed contaminated rapeseed oil; while some showed no symptoms or recovered after developing only transient symptoms, women with particular tissue types (DR3 or DR4) were more likely to develop chronic disease (*Vicario et al., 1982*).

The toxic-oil syndrome, like the eosinophilia-myalgia syndrome, has a number of features which still remain unexplained, but it is clear that the disease depends on genetic and other factors, apart from contact with the toxic agent itself. In other, milder outbreaks of illness caused by contaminated food or environmental pollution, it is even more difficult to detect, diagnose, and trace the origin of reactions which develop insidiously over a period of days, weeks or months. The incidence of clinical reactions to toxins or to contaminated food could, therefore, be higher than is generally realized. There is clearly a need for further research in this area.

A distinction needs to be drawn between such toxic effects and the notion that there is an unspecified type of hypersensitive reaction which cannot be detected by any of the accepted immunological tests. Many of the claims which have caught the attention, or fired the imagination, of journalists have now gone well beyond the limits of dispassionate assessment. In the United States, Rinkel, Randolph and Zeller (1951) and Dickey (1976) attributed a variety of ailments to food allergy, and proposed a number of unproven remedies for their treatment. In the United Kingdom, two books by R. Mackarness [*Not All in the Mind* (1976) and *Chemical Victims* (1980)] presented a disturbing, but uncritical, approach to environmental issues in the modern world. Both books presented a direct approach to the lay reader, but with no attempt to present evidence to the medical profession. Their claims to provide a 'revolutionary approach to the modern epidemics' or 'a startling look at the threat to your health' raised considerable questions concerning their objectivity, especially as the 'modern epidemics' were said to include allergies, headaches, lethargy, obesity, bowel disturbances, depression and other mental illnesses. Perhaps not surprisingly, there has been much professional criticism aimed at those who offer their views to the general public without providing evidence for medical inspection. Nevertheless, the explanations of Mackarness and others proved to be extremely popular with patients who felt that their symptoms had been summarily dismissed, or treated unsympathetically or inadequately by other members of the medical profession.

The Total Allergy Syndrome

The concept of 'total allergy' reached the newspaper headlines some years ago when funds were raised by English well-wishers to purchase treatment for an ill woman who wished to be admitted to an environmentally controlled unit in the United States. The suggestion was that the patient was a very sensitive individual who could not tolerate exposure to the chemical contaminants in our industrial and domestic environment, including petrol fumes and sulphur dioxide in the air we breathe, artificial preservatives in our food and drink, and even the plasticizers which are present in tap water. The remedy was to transfer the patient to an enclosed environment to receive specially prepared food while breathing filtered air. Over a period of a year or so, the concept of 'allergy to the twentieth century' was remarkably in vogue, and many general practitioners found themselves seeing self-diagnosed patients who believed they recognized the condition in themselves. The criteria for making the diagnosis remained unclear, however. The reported symptoms were not those of the severe, multiple allergies which are certainly seen in patients with asthma or eczema, but included weakness, lethargy, faintness, convulsions, black-outs, anginal pain, exaggerated breathing, migraine, disorders of the bowel and bladder, aching joints, and hypersensitivity of the skin. To this list was added the not uncommon symptoms of the hyperventilation syndrome (described in Chapter 2), including symmetrical tingling of the limbs and muscle cramps – symptoms which have now been attributed to the effects of overbreathing, which can lead to carbon dioxide loss and, through the loss of its acidity and ability to dilate blood vessels, to a number of other consequences (*Nixon, 1982; Freeman, 1989*). In the wake of leading articles in the London newspapers *The Observer* and *The Sunday Times*, proposals were made for the setting-up of such environmental units within the British National Health Service – perhaps reflecting the trust which the public places in the suggestions made in newspaper and television reports. The criteria for diagnosing total allergy remained unclear, and the disease has since disappeared from our television screens. By 1990, the patient whose illness first attracted this diagnostic label asserted that her first encounter with those who made that diagnosis was the worst event of her life.

A case for developing environmental units has yet to be made. While it is arguable that filtered air and protection from environmental allergens could be of value in patients with extremely severe asthma and other allergic disorders, the rarity of such cases has meant inevitably that, once a unit of this kind is established, it tends to be used inappropriately for a wide range of other conditions.

Unorthodox Diagnosis and Treatment

There is no problem in diagnosing food reactions in patients who have obvious, immediate reactions to a particular food on several occasions, usually involving swelling of the lips, asthma, skin reactions, or a severe gastrointestinal or other generalized reaction. Although tests involving the administration of food by mouth could be hazardous in very severe cases, for most patients, the only objective way to confirm a clinical food reaction is to give the food by mouth. Tests for the presence of IgE antibodies can provide a measure of support, but the gold standard for the diagnosis of such reactions remains the double-blind placebo-controlled food challenge test (described in Chapter 2).

Claims have been made concerning the use of a number of other diagnostic methods which purport to identify food reactions or other forms of environmental illness to which clinical ecologists apply such terms as 'multiple-chemical sensitivities', 'cerebral allergy', 'chemically induced immune dysregulation', 'twentieth century disease', 'ecological illness', and 'food-and-chemical sensitivities'. Any objective assessment of the validity of such tests must begin by examining the diagnostic criteria which define the disease (*Royal College of Physicians, 1992*). It is apparent that the range of symptoms included in the ecologist's diagnostic criteria are likely to encourage the diagnosis of environmental illness in many patients with unexplained fatigue, depression, other forms of psychiatric illness, obsessional attitudes to health and diet, food fads, or bowel disturbances, all of which may be caused by a variety of important diseases and which can only be treated satisfactorily if appropriately investigated and correctly diagnosed. While some patients with fatigue may well have symptoms following a viral infection, sometimes called post-viral fatigue syndrome, myalgic encephalomyelitis or ME (*Olson et al., 1986a,b; Muir et al., 1991; Lloyd et al., 1990*), others who complain of fatigue have quite different physical or mental problems, including those who 'somatize', which is to say that they feel physically ill when under psychological strain (see p.49). Test results which rely solely on the subjective comments of the patient can often mislead, as in the case of anxious individuals who overbreathe when they recognize a particular test food and, by so doing, provoke symptoms similar to those attributable to food-induced reactions (*Lum, 1981*; see p.20 and Chapter 6).

The clinical ecologist is not alone among the practitioners of alternative medicine in devising diagnostic tests based on the concept of a clinically recognizable 'response' to a virtually unlimited range of environmental agents that produce symptoms which are mainly subjective and not associated with a consistent or characteristic physical sign, pathological abnormality or diagnostic laboratory test (*Magarian, 1982*). The conventional challenge test achieves objectivity by comparing the patient's reaction to a disguised test substance with the response to a similarly disguised harmless placebo. Instead of this method, however, a number of other procedures have been used and claim to be of diagnostic value. These include the injection provocation-neutralization test, cytotoxic blood test, blood count of lymphocyte subsets, and other procedures such as reflexology, iridology, hair analysis and electrokinesis (*Royal College of Physicians, 1992*). With no recourse to the equivalent of a Consumer Protection Act, many vulnerable people are exposed to well publicized claims concerning the value of highly dubious test methods to be carried out on blood, hair, or urine. In other tests, changes may be noted in pulse rate, skin or muscle. These are of little or no value and include:

1. **The pulse test.** This test, in various forms, has persisted from the time it was first described by Coca in 1942. It is based on the belief that a food-allergic patient has an increase in heart rate after ingesting the relevant food. While this is sometimes the case, an increased pulse rate is such a common finding in anxious patients during the course of a challenge test that the method is valueless.

2. **Sublingual provocative food test.** This is based on the theory that the absorption of ingested substances through the mucous membrane under the tongue is sufficient to produce a mild physical reaction. It has been used in conjunction with a form of treatment in which drops of dilute food solutions are placed under the tongue, especially for hay fever (*Scadding & Brostoff, 1986*). A series of studies has shown that the method fails to discriminate between control substances and food extracts (*Caplin, 1973; Breneman et al., 1974; Lehman, 1980a*).

3. **Provocation-neutralization test.** This method has a number of variations, but requires the administration of successively higher doses of a test substance by injection or by sublingual drops until the patient reports the development of any symptom (not necessarily one that has been previously encountered), or until there is an increase in size of a cutaneous weal in those cases in which the substance has been injected. Lower or higher doses are then given serially until symptoms disappear, and this 'neutralizing dose' is then used by the patient for self-treatment.

This test has been reviewed by a Clinical Efficacy Assessment Subcommittee of the American College of Physicians and, subsequently, by the California Medical Association (1986). A further survey of 91 papers on clinical ecology by the American College of Physicians (1989) found no published evidence of its effectiveness which stood up to critical examination. Furthermore, when tests are carried out by placing drops under the tongue, only a single item can be tested at one time. Sequential 10-minute tests can fill an entire day, and a complete series of tests can take several days. Any attempt to reproduce this method must also involve food extracts of poorly defined content, since the chemical composition of food varies. The tests involve a heterogeneous group of patients and make use of vague endpoints which cannot be identified with any certainty (*Hirsch et al., 1981*). In a carefully planned, double-blind study, the response of patients to the recommended test solutions and placebo injections was indistinguishable (*Breneman et al., 1974*). More recent studies have also failed to validate the well publicized claims that have been made for this method (*Jewett et al., 1990; Hunter, 1991*).

4. **Cytotoxic food test.** When Black (*1956*) claimed that the white blood cells of food-allergic patients disintegrate in the presence of food-allergens, he devised a test in which the white blood cells are mixed with extracts of the suspected food on microscope slides, and the number of damaged white cells counted. Lehman (*1980b*) showed that the results of this test varied so greatly from one day to another that it was of no diagnostic value. Its unreliability has been confirmed in an assessment by the American Academy of Allergy and the National Centre for Health Care Technology (*van Metre, 1987*). When blood samples were examined 'blind' by a laboratory specializing in cytotoxic testing, there were gross discrepancies in the reports provided on twinned samples taken from the same individual, and the laboratory reported numerous food allergies both in allergic subjects and in healthy volunteers (*Sethi et al., 1987*).

5. **Diagnosis in environmental control units.** To exclude pollen and other airborne substances that might provoke symptoms, several clinical ecologists have established 'environmental control units' which require filtered air and are entered through double-doors. It has been claimed that, after a period on an elimination diet, food challenge tests and tests with inhaled substances can give more precise results in such an environment. Despite the concern for fine detail with respect to the use of construction materials, such as porcelain, steel, aluminium, ceramic tiles, hard vinyl asbestos tiles and hardwood, the diagnostic endpoints remain subjective.

6. **Hair test.** The use of hair tests has been promulgated as a means of diagnosing food allergy. To those who are invited to send hair samples through the post, the idea may have a certain attractiveness, but the concept has no reasonable basis either in theory or in practice.

While it is true that toxic levels of metals can be detected by hair analysis and, for example, arsenic poisoning can be identified in this way, there is no evidence that hair contains any substances which reflect an allergy to food. When hair samples were tested in the study quoted above (*Sethi et al., 1987*), there were wide discrepancies in the reports provided on duplicate samples taken from the same subjects.

A quite different form of hair analysis is known as 'dowsing', and makes use of a pendulum which is swung over the hair sample. The 'altered swing' which is claimed in cases of food allergy has been used to justify the prescription of grossly unsuitable diets.

7. **Test for *Candida* hypersensitivity syndrome.** *Candida albicans* is a yeast which is normally found in the gastrointestinal tract and can cause thrush infections in individuals with immunological deficiencies or in those who, during a course of antibiotic treatment, have lost the normal bacterial flora that keep the growth of *Candida* in check. Except in the presence of the most gross immunodeficiency, thrush remains a surface infection in the mouth, the vagina or, occasionally, in the fingernails. Its overgrowth in the bowel in antibiotic-associated diarrhoea can occasionally cause problems which, however, can be simply treated by oral nystatin, even when antibiotic treatment is continued at the same time (*Danna et al., 1991*).

These known facts concerning *Candida* contrast with the speculative concept that *Candida* hypersensitivity can depress the immune system and cause an illness with multiple, subjective symptoms even in the absence of any diagnostic evidence. This diagnosis, popularized by the book *The Yeast Connection* (*Crook, 1984*), has provided the clinical ecologist with a further range of treatment methods in patients with persisting symptoms. Oral nystatin may be prescribed, sometimes continuing for months or years, despite the lack of any benefit in a carefully conducted study (*Dismukes et al., 1990*). If this fails, ketoconazole or amphotericin B can be given. The avoidance of sugar is also recommended in the belief that sugars encourage the growth of *Candida*.

As in other instances where sweeping claims have been put forward without adequate supporting evidence, the American Academy of Allergy and Immunology has published a careful report on the position, which found no objective evidence to support the views put forward (*Executive Committee, 1986*). Although allergy to *Candida* can cause allergy (*Gumowski et al., 1987*), currently used allergy tests for *Candida* are so non-specific (*Dhivert et al., 1983*) as to be of no value and cannot justify the attribution of a wide range of symptoms to a '*Candida* hypersensitivity syndrome'. The *Candida* theory remains unsubstantiated.

8. **Other laboratory tests.** It has been well established that immunological mechanisms are involved in classical allergic disorders, such as hay fever and food allergy. This has led to the speculation that immunological changes are responsible for the production of 'environmental illness'. However, attempts to provide a scientific basis for this concept have failed, partly because of the vagueness and lack of definition of what constitutes an environmental illness. Nevertheless, as new tests have become available for complement components, immune complex formation, immunoglobulin levels, immunoglobulin G (IgG) subclass levels, lymphocyte subset counts and the detection of inflammatory mediators in the blood, these have been included in the investigative repertoire for the diagnosis of environmental illness caused by food or chemicals. Despite the suggestion (or the implication) that the most up-to-date tests are being used to confirm the proferred diagnosis, none of these methods has been shown to be of value for this purpose (*American College of Physicians, 1989*).

ALTERNATIVE MEDICAL PRACTICE AND THE PATIENT

Conventional allergists have a limited number of treatments to offer patients with a demonstrable allergic or intolerant response to food or other environmental agents. In cases where the diagnosis is less clear, or where the doctor makes a psychiatric diagnosis which the patient is unwilling to accept, it has become increasingly common – and completely justifiable – for patients to seek alternative views. These views are not always sought from conventional doctors but, when the patient so desires, from practitioners of alternative medicine. Whether the dissatisfied patient is seeking confirmation of a personal self-diagnosis, or a greater degree of patience, sympathy and encouragement from the doctor, the result is by no means always harmful. Acupuncture can sometimes be of benefit in relieving pain; hypnosis has been used to benefit asthmatics who are unduly anxious, and eczema may respond to some herbal remedies (*Royal College of Physicians, 1992*). It should be noted, however, that patients who consult alternative medical practitioners are sometimes encouraged to embark on long courses of treatment, and often develop a lifestyle which is organized around their illness (*Black et al., 1990*). In such a case, a substantial number of patients may persist with the alternative medical doctor's treatment even when it is very protracted and the symptoms respond only transiently or not at all. The danger then lies in the possible failure to detect an illness which requires urgent treatment or, in some cases, the neglect of a major degree of depression which carries the risk of suicide. There are also dangers in following methods of treatment which involve unhealthy diets, reinforce obsessional behaviour, or encourage social isolation.

Vulnerable people should be aware of the many (and expensive) pitfalls for those who accept methods of treatment which are not validated. Even the suggestion that herbal remedies are, at least, harmless does not stand up to examination. In addition to the fatalities caused by penny royal and other abortifacient herbs, and the kidney damage caused by 'organic germanium' used as a food supplement, there are reports of liver damage caused by mistletoe (*Penn, 1983*) and by the herbal remedies called 'Kalms' and 'Neuralax' (*MacGregor et al., 1989*). Some traditional Asian herbal remedies can cause lead and arsenic poisoning (*Aslam et al., 1979; Mitchell-Heggs et al., 1990*). Herbal medicines may also be combined with potentially toxic conventional drugs (including corticosteroids) without disclosure on the label (*Penn, 1986*).

Some of the test methods used by alternative medical practitioners have already been listed, especially those which have been most commonly applied in diagnosing food allergy. A number of other ingeniously named methods are used, often involving elaborate explanations and a ritual form of test procedure, sometimes combined with the use of impressive 'black-box' apparatus, none of which have any scientific validity:

a. The Vega machine measures electrical conductivity over acupuncture points and the patient holds a hand electrode to complete the circuit. Movements of a needle in response to the addition of a test substance are said to identify allergens.

b. Applied kinesiology has been claimed to detect the induction of muscle weakness by allergens, which are either held in a sample bottle or placed under the tongue (*Kenyon, 1986*).

c. Unsubstantiated claims have also been made for an 'auriculo-cardiac reflex' method.

Other methods continue to be investigated despite a lack of convincing evidence. Acupuncture has a traditional use in the relief of pain, possibly because the body's own pain-relieving mechanisms are stimulated. Acupuncture has also been used in Chinese traditional medicine for the treatment of disease, through the location of hundreds of acupuncture points and their identification with different organs of the body. Its use in asthma has been proposed (*Kleijnen et al., 1991*), but remains unproven. No other evidence exists for its value in the treatment of allergy.

Two other methods, enzyme-potentiated desensitization (*Fell & Brostoff, 1990*) and homoeopathy (*Reilly et al, 1986*) have been the subject of poorly substantiated analyses claiming efficacy.

Diagnoses Which Can Be Missed

Most of the problems connected with the inappropriate diagnosis of food allergy lie in the patient mismanagement that follows because the correct diagnosis has been missed. This is especially true of patients with psychiatric problems. Despite the change in attitudes which have reduced the stigma attached to such a diagnosis, many people feel a strong need to attribute such symptoms as fatigue, weakness, nausea or headaches to a physical, rather than a psychological, cause. In some cultures, healers conform to the patient's diagnosis of a physical, rather than an emotional, disorder (*Mechamic & Kleinman, 1980*). The effect of such an approach is not known.

Patients who somatize have already been referred to. It has been estimated that 60% of patients who present themselves to primary care physicians because of problems concerned with psychosocial distress complain repeatedly of physical (somatic) symptoms (*Cummings & Vanden Bos, 1981*). This somatization is probably the most common form taken by mental disorders (*Murphy, 1989*), which may help to explain the vulnerability of patients to newly popularized explanations of their illness and to the use of unproven or even fraudulent treatments based on a misdiagnosis of physical illness (*Stewart, 1990*).

Even in psychiatric illness, however, the symptoms may have a physiological basis and the doctor who is merely dismissive may do the patient no service. Individuals who expect to have an adverse reaction — even to a harmless placebo — have been shown to develop changes in pulse rate and other physiological changes. Similarly, those who experience pain relief after acupuncture are having a physiological response — in this case, involving the release of natural pain-relieving substances within their own bodies. Patients who expect an unpleasant reaction to a food or other external agent who overbreathe can also induce an excessive loss of carbon dioxide in the breath and, by upsetting the acid-base balance of the blood, can provoke giddiness, weakness, tingling, a racing pulse and even a loss of consciousness. These are features of the hyperventilation syndrome, which is common and often unaccompanied by any other physical illness (Table 3.1). Not surprisingly, patients with symptoms of this kind, who feel they have been given no adequate explanation, may seek other opinions and may find comfort if they are offered alternative medical diagnoses. Among the most frequent diagnostic labels given in such cases, Stewart (1990) includes environmental hypersensitivity disorder, candidiasis hypersensitivity syndrome, chronic fatigue, and food allergy.

In spite of the evidence of a large psychiatric component in many instances, this is not true of all, and the need to exclude physical disease has already been mentioned. In patients with a history of postinfective lethargy and evidence of glandular fever, persisting symptoms have been recorded for periods of up to 3 years (*Tobi et al., 1982*) and chronic (postviral) fatigue has received increasing recognition (*Royal College of Physicians, 1992*). In some, however, the interaction between physical and psychological factors can be difficult to unravel.

Cathebras *et al. (1991)* investigated 20 patients in whom other

Table 3.1 Frequency of the hyperventilation syndrome among patients referred to hospital

Type of medical practice	Incidence (%)
Gastroenterology (500 consecutive cases)	5.8
Cardiology clinic	6.0
1000 consecutive new outpatients	10.7

(Freeman, 1989)

causes of fatigue had been excluded and found that, in 10 of them, the tiredness began with a probable infection. Sixteen of the 20 had a clearly diagnosable psychiatric illness, and extensive investigations were unhelpful. Of the 19 patients followed for 2–4 months, 14 recovered and 5 were still symptomatic.

CONCLUSION

A number of health problems have arisen as the result of environmental pollution. There have also been instances in which the chemical contamination of water, cooking oil, flour and tinned food have led to outbreaks of disease. A few sensitive individuals do react to foods or food additives in quantities that cause no harm in the majority of the population.

An awareness of these problems should be coupled by a rejection of the sensationalism and exaggeration which have led to notions of 'allergy to the twentieth century' and to the marketing of well-publicized methods of diagnosis and treatment which cannot be shown to be of any value. Where the diagnosis is incorrect, alternative medical treatments may not only be unnecessarily restrictive or nutritionally inadequate, but can lead to the neglect of undiagnosed illness. It should be added that, like the public at large, purchasers of National Health services and medical insurance agencies should be warned against paying for expensive tests or treatments which cannot be validated.

CHAPTER

—4—

Physiology of Digestion

BASIC FUNCTIONS OF THE GUT

The essential function of the digestive process is to break food down into nutrients which can then be absorbed and reassembled by the body while eliminating infective agents and toxic substances. The body achieves this by moving food through the gastrointestinal tract, thus exposing it to the action of enzymes and mixing it with various secretions. In due course, the digested components are absorbed across the mucosal barriers, allowing entry into the portal vein (and hence to the liver for processing) and also to the lymphatic vessels. Food intolerance can result from failures of either this digestive sequence of events or of the associated mechanisms which serve to discriminate between a nutrient and a hazardous substance that is to be rejected.

The process begins with chewing and the mixing of food with saliva, which contributes to the breakdown of starch, producing maltose as the principal product. Once it is swallowed, food passes rapidly through the oesophagus to be acted upon in the stomach and small intestine by the secretions produced by the stomach itself, the pancreas and the biliary apparatus. The stomach acts, first, as a secreting organ, producing acid and protein-digesting enzymes in the form of pepsinogens, which become activated to pepsins. The stomach then acts as a muscular mixing chamber and, finally, as a reservoir in which, under the influence of enzymes in a highly acid medium, food is progressively liquidized. As this liquidizing process continues, there is a slow rate of emptying into the small bowel. This usually continues for 1–2 hours after a standard meal, feeding the small intestine with partly digested food mixtures for further processing and absorption. The stomach also produces a glycoprotein (intrinsic factor) which helps the absorption of vitamin B_{12} in the ileum, and the lower end of the stomach releases gastrin, a hormone which helps to regulate further activity in the stomach, pancreas, and rest of the bowel.

After the stomach pepsins have begun to hydrolyse proteins, the digestive process is continued in the first 100 cm of the small intestine, mainly under the influence of the enzymes secreted by the pancreas which reduce proteins to small amino acids that persist either singly or in small chains. These enzymes are not secreted continuously. Their release, and the flow of bile, are both stimulated by the arrival of nutrients in the duodenum and the release of the peptide hormone cholecystokinin. Pancreatic lipase and esterase enzymes begin the digestion of fats by their hydrolysing effects, and the detergent action of bile salts then aids their physical dispersion into water-soluble mixtures.

It is in this same region of the small intestine that most of the absorption of nutrients occurs after having been further broken down by a number of brush-border enzymes. The brush border represents the margin between the cells lining the intestine and the intestinal contents. The brush-border enzymes are globular proteins attached to the cell surface by protein stalks. They include at least three peptidases, which continue the breakdown of proteins into amino acids, and also lactase, sucrase and isomaltase, which break down further the partially digested carbohydrates — now mostly in the form of disaccharides and other sugars, and usually including substantial amounts of maltose derived from starch.

The absorptive surface of the small intestine is extraordinarily convoluted with a surface area totalling several hundred square metres. Hair-like structures known as villi are covered by lining cells called enterocytes together with a few scattered lymphocytes. The important absorptive cell is the enterocyte which has a surface formed of even finer hair-like structures (microvilli) (Fig. 4.1) covered by a lipid membrane from which peptidases, disaccharide-splitting enzymes and other mucosal enzymes protrude.

The terminal part of the small intestine and the colon are involved primarily in reclaiming the fluid and electrolytes secreted during the

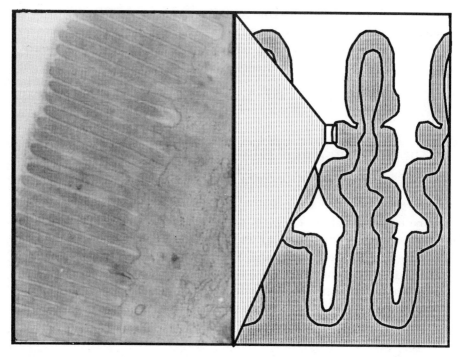

Fig. 4.1
Surface of the enterocyte: (left) Low-power electronmicrograph showing microvilli from the middle portion of a normal villus. (right) The large absorptive surface of the enterocyte is apparent. By courtesy of Dr A.D. Phillips, Queen Elizabeth Hospital for Children, London, UK.

digestive process. Considerable quantities of fluid are processed in this way. Apart from the 1–2 litres of water which, on average, are ingested daily, 8–10 litres of fluid enter the gut in the form of secretions, almost all of which is reabsorbed, mainly in the small intestine. Very little fluid is therefore lost with a normal stool, which may contain as little as 0.1 litre of water.

The movement of contents through different parts of the bowel is summarized in Table 4.1. After 2–6 hours in the small intestine, the colon moves the residual material towards the rectum over a period of 12 hours or so, during which there are prolonged periods of mixing and brief periods of movement. This activity takes place under the combined influence of the nervous tissue network, and a number of locally released hormones that, among them, regulate the movement in the bowel, the secretion of water, electrolytes, mucus and enzymes, the

Table 4.1 Movement of contents through the gastrointestinal tract

Segment	Time of passage
Oesophagus	4– 8 seconds
Stomach	1– 2 hours
Small intestine	2– 6 hours
Colon	12–24 hours

contraction of the gall bladder, the mixing of food and bile, the release of other hormones, and intestinal absorption itself. Details of the hormonal and nervous control mechanisms, and of the enzymic digestion of food and its absorption, have been well reviewed by others (*Bloom et al., 1987; Parsons, 1987*).

The mechanisms which are capable of digesting food also have a protective role. Although some bacteria are capable of resisting acid peptic digestion, they may nevertheless be unable to penetrate the mucous glycoproteins which protect the gastric mucosa and help to prevent the attachment of infective agents. If bacteria do penetrate, they may be recognized as foreign (antigenic) substances and, as such, provoke a protective immune response.

It is generally true that proteins, starches, fat and even vitamins are broken down into simpler molecules before absorption can occur. Even in health, however, some intact molecules can be absorbed and are detectable in the blood circulation while, in diseases associated with damage to the wall of the bowel, this passage of intact food molecules across the bowel wall may be sufficiently antigenic to provoke the body to produce food-binding proteins – that is, antibodies – in significantly higher quantities than are seen in health.

The very complex mechanisms which regulate the motility, secretory and absorptive functions of the bowel involve a local network of nervous tissues in the wall of the gut that is controlled by the autonomic nervous system. They are also influenced by locally released hormones and various other hormones, which enter the bloodstream and can also modify gastrointestinal tone and motility. The autonomic nervous system, the regulating hormones and the digestive enzymes share control over the process of digestion, the absorption of nutrients and the elimination of residue. There are also regulatory mechanisms for the immunological reactions that provide the body's chief form of protection against foreign substances that either penetrate the skin or the membranes lining the lungs or the gastrointestinal tract. These reactions can be either induced or suppressed according to circumstances. While soluble food components are tolerated, bacteria and other substances which reach the lumen of the bowel may provoke a battery of protective responses which will wash away or destroy the invader.

Role of the Digestive Enzymes

The breakdown of food prior to its absorption involves numerous enzymic processes and a variety of protein enzymes, which are either secreted into the lumen of the bowel or attached to the surface of cells (Fig. 4.2). The production, action and recycling of digestive enzymes follows a regular pattern. In the duodenum, pancreatic secretions neutralize the acid products of the stomach, and there is an outpouring of water (approximately 1 litre per day) containing sodium bicarbonate. The pancreatic secretions reach a peak within 45 minutes after a meal and continue at a high rate until the duodenum has emptied. Approximately 8 grams of enzyme protein are secreted daily into a mixture which consists mainly of hydrolases which are capable of breaking down protein (proteases), fat (lipases) and starch. In the presence of bile, fat breakdown occurs rapidly, thereby producing free fatty acids and monoglycerides.

Role of Bile

Bile is formed in liver cells and bile ducts, and is stored and concentrated in the gall bladder from which it is expelled when food enters the small intestine. The secretion of bile plays an important role and includes bile acids and bile salts which are related to cholesterol and are responsible for the solubilization of lipids. By maintaining water-soluble aggregates (micelles), they help poorly soluble fat

Fig. 4.2
Role of enzymes in digestion: 8 g of digestive enzymes are secreted daily to break down food protein, fat and carbohydrates before reabsorption can take place. The breakdown products after absorption are also exposed to enzymes in the blood and liver.

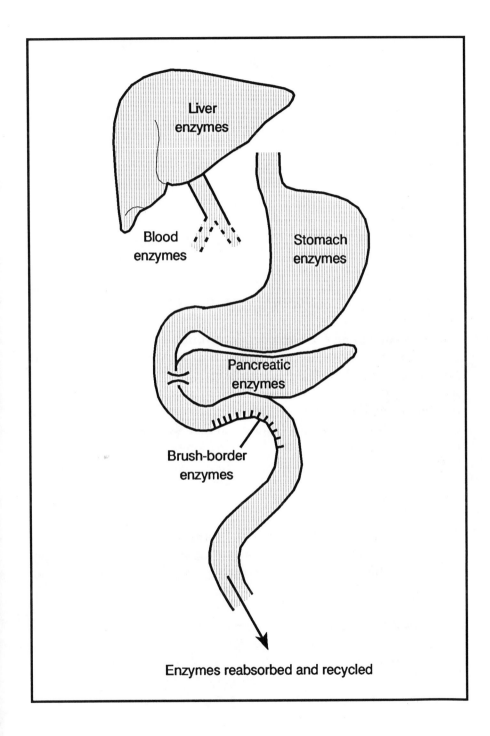

products to diffuse through the fluid layer which covers the enterocytes and thus play a vital part in facilitating the absorption of dietary lipids and fat-soluble vitamins.

The processes whereby the digestive fluids, enzymes and bile are reabsorbed and recycled have formed the subject of numerous studies. The economy exhibited by the digestive system is remarkable. Conjugated bile acids are reabsorbed in the final portion of the small bowel and travel through the portal blood to the liver, where they are taken up into the liver cells and re-excreted. This process functions so well that the total bile-acid pool has been shown to circulate at least twice per meal in experimental studies in humans. Only 2% of the bile salts are lost in the faeces or broken down.

MUCOSAL IMMUNITY

The mucosal immune tissue provides a discriminating system which adapts quickly to new circumstances. It is capable of accepting both food antigens and harmless bacteria. Even when a low-grade response to food antigens occurs, the absorption of nutritious substances is not prevented. At the same time, the mucosal tissue reacts vigorously to potentially damaging microorganisms and parasites. In this way, it can eliminate infection and, by the dissemination of sensitized cells to other sites of the body, mount longer-lasting protection to prevent reinfection at other points of entry into the body.

In many severe diseases of the stomach or intestine, digestive functions remain remarkably normal, and immunological reactions to foods are unaffected. While simple restrictions in diet may be necessary in intestinal disease – a low-fat diet in patients with fat malabsorption, or a low-residue diet for patients with an intestinal stricture – food-intolerant reactions or disordered immune responses to foods are relatively uncommon. The intestinal tract, even in health, contains a range of substances that are all capable of stimulating the immune system when absorbed unchanged. These include bacterial breakdown products, food proteins and complex carbohydrates. These substances are normally broken down by intestinal enzymes, but a failure of this process and absorption of the intact, antigenic substances could lead to a number of immunologically mediated diseases. As a barrier to the absorption of harmful substances, the mucous secretions, lining cells of the mucosa, and gut-associated lymphoid tissue all have a central role.

The most important cell of the lymphoid system is the lymphocyte, a cell capable of either reacting directly with specific foreign substances to which the body has become sensitized, or producing various types of chemical antidotes (antibodies) which are capable of circulating in the bloodstream or diffusing into the tissues. The intestine of an adult contains around 800 billion (8×10^{10}) lymphocytes, making it by far the largest lymphoid organ in the body. This compares with approximately 200 billion in the bone marrow, spleen and lymph nodes combined. The most prominent component of the gut-associated lymphoid tissue (GALT) consists of specialized areas known as Peyer's patches, each of which contains approximately 30–40 groups of cells clustered in follicles. These cells are mostly lymphocytes of the directly reacting variety (T cells), and of the type capable of producing antibodies (B cells). In addition to these concentrated patches, there are also many smaller nodules and scattered lymphocytes among the lining layers of the intestine.

Lymphocytes can be activated in various ways – by specialized microfold cells (Fig. 4.3), by large cells (macrophages) present in the bloodstream, or by finely branching cells called dendrocytes present within the tissues. Lymphocytes which have been activated within the Peyer's patch are absorbed into the lymph-carrying channels (lymphatic system). They then pass through lymph nodes to reach the circulating bloodstream and finally 'seed' themselves back into the walls of the intestine at even more sites, where they are able to respond immediately to any further encounters with the same antigen. Lymphocytes also seed themselves at other mucosal sites, notably, within the breast and in the airways of the lung (Fig. 4.4). In addition to the local surface protection which this can provide, the lactating mother can donate protective antibody to her offspring through her milk.

Both T and B lymphocytes can circulate and re-seed but, for most B lymphocytes, it is not the cells themselves that relocate to other parts of the body, but their antibody products. Antibodies are specifically adapted molecules with a basic immunoglobulin structure (Fig. 4.5) which are able to bind to foreign material and also form attachments at

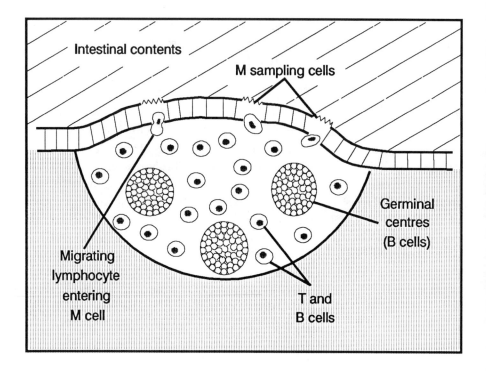

Fig. 4.3

The Peyer's patch as a sampling organ: Microfold (M) sampling cells can bring foreign protein into contact with lymphocytes.

the other end of their molecule, thereby linking the foreign material to various other types of protective cells or inflammatory proteins (complement). This form of linkage triggers a reaction capable of damaging, destroying or engulfing the foreign material; specialized, inflammation-mediating mast cells can be activated by such a process (Fig. 4.6).

This combination of different mechanisms provides the body with in-depth protection. The intestinal wall is covered by a mucous layer, which behaves like an antiseptic coat of paint, and contains antibodies of the immunoglobulin A (IgA) and immunoglobulin M (IgM) classes. Of the two other important classes of immunoglobulin, IgG (Fig. 4.5) circulates in the blood, but can also diffuse into the tissues. Immunoglobulin E (IgE) acts indirectly by adhering to the surface of

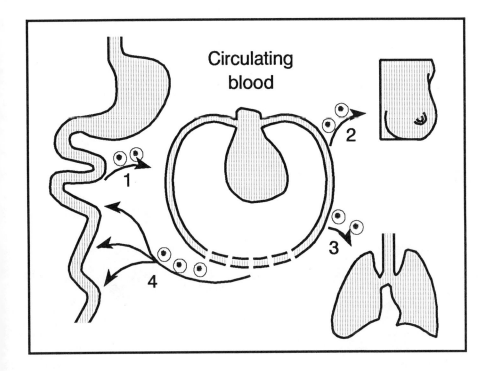

Fig. 4.4
Migration and dissemination of sensitized lymphocytes: 1, Lymphocytes sensitized in the intestine reach the circulating bloodstream; 2–4, Recirculated lymphocytes 'home in' to the breast, lungs and widespread sites in the intestine, thereby 'seeding' populations of protective cells throughout the body.

scattered mast cells, which are found below the skin and mucous surfaces of the body in close contact with nerve endings. Mast cells in the intestine differ in some respects from those below the skin, but both types possess specialized high-affinity receptors on their surfaces to which IgE molecules attach. When a foreign molecule makes contact with two adjacent IgE molecules on the surface of a mast cell, it triggers the release of histamine and other stored substances capable of provoking inflammation; it also provokes the mast cell to synthesize a number of arachidonic acid metabolites on its surface, in particular, leukotrienes and prostaglandins. The release of these substances is characteristic of an allergic response. It should be noted that mast cells

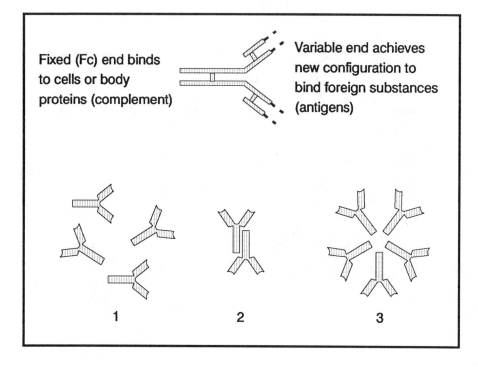

Fig. 4.5

Basic structure of immunoglobulin (Ig): There is a fixed end and a variable end. The reconfigured Ig has the ability to react with specific foreign substances, and is now an **antibody.** *The basic structure of the different classes of Ig are: 1, IgG and IgE; 2, IgA (a dimer with two linked molecules); 3, IgM (a pentamer with five linked molecules).*

can also be activated in other ways, for example by histamine-releasing foods (*Anderson & Sogn, 1984*) or when stimulated by the nervous system (*Stead et al, 1989*).

Foreign substances that penetrate the mucous barrier and the lining cells of the intestinal tract thus meet further obstacles before

Fig. 4.6

Activation of mast cells: 1, B cell synthesizes IgE antibody to a foreign protein; 2, IgE antibody attaches to mast cell surface; 3, A foreign protein (antigen) crosslinks two IgE molecules on mast cell surface; 4, Preformed granules containing histamine, enzymes and inflammatory substances are discharged. There is also the release of newly formed chemicals and chemical messengers from the cell membrane.

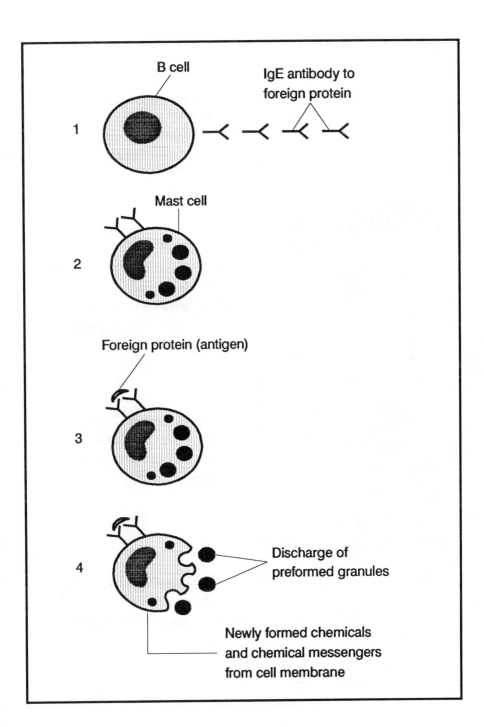

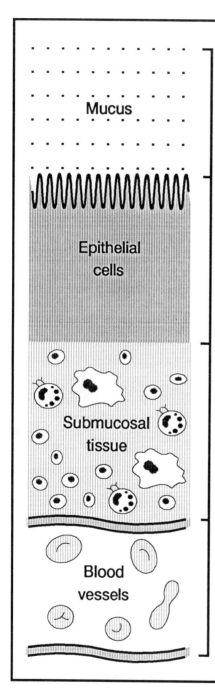

Mucus

Prevents attachment of infective agents

Binds toxic substances

Contains antibodies and digestive enzymes

Epithelial cells

Physical barrier to large molecules and bacteria

Surmounted by a brush border containing digestive enzymes

Submucosal tissue

Contains further immunological defences - mast cells, lymphocytes, macrophages (scavenger cells)

Blood vessels

Blood cells (including protective white cells)

Plasma (including antibodies and enzymes)

penetrating the body's in-depth defences (Fig. 4.7). The discharge of mast cells or the triggering of sensitized lymphocytes provide a substantial capacity for provoking inflammation and all of the features of an allergic response, while reactions with immunoglobulins in the tissues can lead to further inflammatory effects which, in turn, are capable of being amplified.

Amplifying Mechanisms

As an example of the way in which penetration of a few molecules can provoke a crescendo of inflammatory changes, the enzymes known collectively as 'complement' hold a special place. These enzymes are activated in sequence, with each complement component (C) triggering the next series of components, from C1 to C9. When antibody combines with antigen, C1 may become attached, one of the ways in which the sequence may begin. The release of a series of inflammatory substances leads to an increase in the permeability of blood vessels, the attraction of white blood cells and the involvement of a variety of migrating cells, including T cells and a subpopulation of 'killer' cells. T cells can infiltrate virtually all tissues and, by releasing chemicals known as lymphokines, can attract further inflammatory cells to the region.

Immune Responses to Ingested Substances

These protective mechanisms are important to the understanding of food allergy, as allergy is 'immunity gone wrong'. The protective function is well illustrated when B lymphocytes are sensitized in the intestine of a nursing mother. These sensitized cells circulate and home in, not only to the gut, but also to breast tissue (Fig. 4.4). There they can produce the surface-protecting IgA antibodies that defend the suckling infant from any bacteria which may have previously penetrated into the mother's body or may even have caused a bout of gastroenteritis. Each class of antibodies acts differently, however. IgA has a structure which is resistant to digestion and is, therefore, ideally suited to its protective role within the bowel, where it diffuses into the mucous secretions of the intestine, and prevents colonization by microbes or penetration of antigenic substances through the intestinal wall. In comparison to IgA,

---

Fig. 4.7
Intestinal defences in depth.

IgE with its capacity to sensitize mast cells provides a second line of defence. IgG and IgM differ yet again; both circulate within the bloodstream, but IgM is also present in mucous secretions, while the smaller molecules of IgG are able to diffuse into tissue.

In most circumstances, the body distinguishes between potentially harmful agents, which trigger the protective immune mechanisms, and digested food, which does not. When the soluble antigens of food first reach lymphoid tissue – in infancy and childhood – they are recognized as harmless and induce a long-lasting form of 'oral tolerance' through the effect of suppressor T cells. This type of tolerance is most easily induced in infancy and early childhood, at a time when new foods are most frequently encountered. This is also the most common time for things to go wrong and for allergy to develop, particularly when one or both parents of the child have themselves inherited a tendency to develop allergic reactions.

Antigenic foods

Most of the foods which are capable of acting as antigens and provoking an immunological reaction are proteins or glycoproteins. Codfish protein and a number of others have been isolated and analysed in detail. The more reactive proteins in milk and egg have a molecular weight of 10,000 to 50,000, but there is no absolute rule which limits their size or molecular structure. The vigour of the reaction against them may depend in part on their similarity or differences from human proteins – one of the most reactive proteins for cow's milk-allergic infants is beta-lactoglobulin, which is not present in large quantities, but has the distinction of being the only type of protein which is absent from human milk (see Chapter 8).

Once an allergic reaction to a protein has developed, there may be cross-reactions with similar proteins from other sources, for example, between the albumen of egg white, the proteins of egg yolk, and the eggs of other birds. The resistance of a protein to cooking may also determine its antigenic potential. Proteins of milk or egg are denatured by cooking and are sometimes tolerated by allergic subjects in their cooked form. Peanut proteins are relatively heat stable, however, so these nuts can cause as much trouble roasted as raw. Food antigens are considered further in Chapter 6.

Biogenic Amines

There are many clinical reactions to food that mimic allergic reactions but do not have an immunological cause. Urticarial weals of the skin or asthmatic reactions may develop, or there may be other physical events indistinguishable in symptoms or appearance from true allergy. The term 'pseudoallergic reaction' is sometimes used for this type of response; Moneret-Vautrin (1983) used the term 'false food allergy'. Our understanding of these reactions is still in its infancy, but the chemical (pharmacological) effect of biologically powerful amine substances (biogenic amines) provides a good example. As far as these substances are concerned, at least three major mechanisms are involved:

1. An abnormally high intake of biogenic amines such as histamine and tyramine, or their synthesis in the gut by bacteria;

2. An abnormal release of histamine and other chemical mediators from mast cells, sometimes triggered by foods such as shellfish, strawberries and alcohol (de Weck, 1984);

3. An abnormal effect, produced by drugs or components of food, which interferes with the enzymes normally capable of digesting amines, or interferes with the part of the nervous system that, by regulating intestinal activity, affects absorption.

It has been estimated that less than 3% of patients with recurrent skin weals (chronic urticaria) have true food allergy, but that non-allergic reactions to food occur in 40% of cases. Pseudoallergic reactions are therefore much more common than true food allergy. A substantial number of patients with urticarial reactions also have abdominal symptoms, including pain and intermittent diarrhoea.

Biologically active amines are normal constituents of many foods and arise mainly from the decarboxylation of amino acids. They may also develop during normal cooking and storage. In addition, they may be synthesized by microorganisms in the intestine or formed as a result of enzymatic changes in the body. Some examples include histamine, which is derived from histidine, and tyramine, which is produced from tyrosine. The largest amounts of histamine and tyramine are found in fermented foods, such as cheese, alcoholic drinks, tinned fish and fish products, sauerkraut, pork and sausage.

Some of these foods contain enough histamine to raise the histamine level of the urine after they have been consumed (Feldman, 1983). Badly stored mackerel and tuna can contain added amounts of histamine produced by marine bacteria. Such foods can cause short, but potentially severe, episodes of flushed skin, diarrhoea and vomiting, sometimes with skin weals, asthma and shock. Although resembling allergic reactions, they are, in fact, caused by absorbed amines. Cereal grains and various vegetables also contain diamines and catecholamines which have potential biological effects.

In general, the effects produced by these substances vary considerably. If it penetrates as far as the bloodstream, histamine may cause flushing by dilating the blood vessels. It can also increase capillary permeability, and cause constriction of the smooth muscle of the lung bronchi and intestine. When histamine is infused into the bloodstream experimentally, it has been seen to stimulate gastric secretion and, above certain levels, the pulse rate increases, headache occurs, and blood pressure falls. Still higher levels have led to asthma and the possibility of cardiac arrest.

Tyramine causes the arteries to constrict, stimulates the release of more adrenaline from nerve endings, and has been reported to release histamine and prostaglandins from mast cells, thus causing headaches and skin symptoms (Maga, 1978). Foods containing tyramine have excited interest because they were shown to produce hypertensive crises and episodes of severe headache in patients who were taking monoamine oxidase inhibitors as treatment for depression (Blackwell et al., 1967). Of the foods taken before the onset of a reaction, cheese was found to contain up to 1.42 mg/g of tyramine; yeast extracts, such as 'Marmite', contained a similar amount as well as some histamine; and pickled herring contained 3 mg/g of tyramine. Blackwell noted that tyramine or other pressor substances were also present in alcoholic beverages, chocolate and, possibly, cream, milk, fish, meat and broad beans. As little as 6 mg of tyramine by mouth was able to cause a reaction.

Hanington (1983) studied 500 migraine sufferers who were selected because each thought their attacks were sometimes linked with certain foods. The foods avoided for this reason were chocolate in three-quarters of those studied, cheese and dairy products in almost one-half and, in descending order, citrus fruits, alcoholic drinks, fried fatty food, vegetables (especially onions), tea and coffee, meat (especially pork) and seafood. Because of the similarity of these patients' list to those foods found to provoke hypertension and headaches in Blackwell's study, Hanington suggested that tyramine and other monoamines could be a common factor. While capsules containing 125 mg of tyramine hydrochloride provoked migraine attacks significantly more frequently than lactose capsules, Hanington considered that tyramine was not the only amine involved in dietary migraine. She noted that cheese and alcoholic beverages also contained significant amounts of betaphenylethylamine (BPEA) and histamine, citrus fruits contained octopamine and synephrine and, while chocolate contained no tyramine, it did contain BPEA in amounts found to provoke migraine attacks.

Despite the evidence of many patients that there is a close relationship between the taking of foods such as cheese, chocolate or wine and the onset of migraine attacks, Hanington's observations have not been clearly confirmed. In the study of the biochemical effects of vasoactive amines, the variability of migraine, and its dependence on potentiating factors such as stress, hypoglycaemia or hormonal changes, has made it a difficult subject to evaluate. It will be discussed further in Chapter 6.

Defence against amines

When injected into the bloodstream, 1 mg of histamine is more than enough to cause side-effects, whereas 200–500 mg of histamine can be instilled into the small intestine without causing symptoms. This is partly because the histamine is inactivated by the mucoproteins secreted by the lining cells of the intestinal tract. This inactivating process can be interfered with by other amines (putresceine and cadaverine) which also bind strongly to mucoproteins. When food is taken which contains putresceine and cadaverine, more histamine can therefore be absorbed. Further defences are also present, and most of the histamine is degraded by the intestinal enzyme diamine oxidase as it is absorbed across the bowel wall. As putresceine and cadaverine have a high affinity for diamine oxidase, they can also interfere with the inactivation of histamine by this enzyme.

The liver enzyme methyl transferase provides yet another protective barrier. Moneret-Vautrin (1983) showed that, when 70-100 mg of histamine was infused into the intestine through a tube, some of it penetrated as far as the liver, but not beyond. It was not until 180 mg was instilled that histamine levels rose substantially in the circulating blood. Subsequent studies demonstrated that much higher blood levels could occur after the intestinal infusion of histamine in subjects with chronic urticaria than in those with other types of urticaria or in normal subjects. In some cases, urticarial reactions following food intake may therefore reflect a pseudoallergic response provoked by increased histamine absorption, rather than by the release of histamine during a sensitivity reaction. In keeping with this view, Moneret-Vautrin (1991) found that, after histamine was instilled into the intestine, 25 out of 42 patients with chronic urticaria developed itching (pruritus), urticaria or headaches.

What appears to be a simple skin reaction in a sensitive person may therefore depend on several factors, including the amount of amine contained in a food, the permeability of the bowel wall, an increase in the release of histamine (sometimes, but not always, caused by allergy), or interference with the synthesis or release of the enzymes involved in histamine breakdown – for example, when the liver is damaged in acute hepatitis. It has been suggested that the breakdown enzymes themselves can be inhibited by sodium nitrite or other food additives, or by alcohol, antibiotics or other drugs (Moneret-Vautrin, 1991).

While histamine has been the most intensively studied biogenic amine, it is likely that an inability to metabolize tyramine can also cause symptoms. In particular, it is known that tyramine can provoke headaches (Sandler et al., 1970) and, in patients who are taking drugs that interfere with the breakdown of tyramine, headaches and a sharp rise in blood pressure can be caused by eating cheese, which contains tyramine in large amounts.

DISORDERS OF INTESTINAL MOTILITY

The ways in which the stomach and intestine react to noxious substances is fairly stereotyped. The classical response to agents which the body fails to recognize as food – that is, an increase in motility of the bowel leading to vomiting or diarrhoea – is the response to all potentially harmful material. This has the effect of ejecting unwanted material and pouring out fluid in large quantities in what amounts to a washing-away process. The overall effect is similar to that seen in the nose, where sneezing and an outpouring of fluid provides a single type of response to a variety of triggering agents, which can be as different as an infecting virus or a grain of pollen in a hay-fever sufferer. Despite the apparent similarity in the response to infective and non-infective agents, however, there are important differences; these are illustrated by the response to rotavirus infections of infancy (see Chapter 6).

The distinction between a normal physiological process and the disordered function of disease is not always easy to make. Clinical complaints range in severity from an overperception of normal peristalsis and wind to the prostrating colic associated with an obstructed bowel. Not surprisingly, there is no single explanation for the 'irritable bowel syndrome', wherein the patient complains of abdominal pain, bloating, constipation or diarrhoea (or an alternation between the two) in the absence of evidence of organic disease. Thompson and Heaton (1980) found that 30% of apparently healthy, uncomplaining British adults admitted to bowel disturbances similar to those which, in other individuals, aroused sufficient concern to necessitate a visit to a hospital clinic. Irritable bowel symptoms account for at least one-third, and sometimes two-thirds, of the hospital consultations for gastrointestinal symptoms, and women are affected twice as frequently as men. In some patients, there is evidence of a link with a specific intolerance to one or more specific foods (*Alun Jones, 1985*).

Disordered intestinal motility may be a presenting symptom in virtually any condition in which unabsorbed food residues reach the lower bowel, where they become subject to bacterial fermentation with the production of acid residues and gases. It follows that irritable bowel symptoms provoked by wheat bran, a lack of the lactose-digesting enzyme lactase, and fatty diarrhoea due to coeliac disease may have a number of features in common. These conditions are considered further in Chapter 6.

CONCLUSION

The anatomical features of the bowel emphasize the complexity of its role. As the largest lymphoid organ in the body, it plays a major part in protecting the body against the toxic and contaminating substances which gain entry in the company of food. The primary function of the bowel is, however, the digestion and absorption of the food itself. To achieve this, it is regulated by a network of nervous tissue and by the largest output of hormones in the body. Some of the digested food components are then used to produce energy, while others are assimilated and resynthesized to maintain the body's own tissues.

The mechanisms which control and regulate the uptake of the

intestinal contents can be disrupted or influenced by factors which interfere with the intestinal flora, the gastric barrier, mucus release from goblet cells, the action of enzymes, the intact structure and motility of the bowel, or filtration and detoxification by the liver. In each of these and in other contributory ways, there is always a possibility of disruption or damage to the point at which there may be a disturbance of function or provocation of symptoms. When the body's surface defences are breached, there is also the prospect of an immunological and inflammatory response which may be protective, but may also be a cause of clinical symptoms or disease.

The origin of any adverse reaction to food can thus depend on several different components. Indeed, it is sometimes the combined effect of several factors which determines the clinical outcome. This may help to explain how clinical recovery can sometimes occur while some adverse factors persist – for example, an enzyme deficiency or an IgE antibody response. In its ability to adapt to such adverse circumstances, the body often shows a remarkable resilience.

CHAPTER

—5—

Mechanisms of Food Intolerance

Food reactions are most easily recognized when they involve the rapid, dramatic onset of severe symptoms – for example, when there is an immediate swelling of the lips or mouth, or when there is a generalized skin reaction, vomiting, and a sudden fall in blood pressure. These are characteristic features of the altered reactivity which has acquired the name of anaphylaxis.

The association of anaphylaxis with changes in the function of the immune system was first recognized early in this century, when reactions to foreign protein, insect venom and certain foods were shown to follow this pattern. In 1921, Prausnitz and Küstner carried out studies which showed that the substance responsible for this altered reactivity was present in serum. They took serum from a fish-sensitive subject (Küstner) and injected it into the skin of a non-sensitive recipient (Prausnitz). The next day, a fish extract was injected into the same site and, as a control, the fish extract was also injected into an area of skin which had not been infiltrated with Küstner's serum. The fish extract provoked the development of a weal, but only in the area of skin which had been pretreated with Küstner's serum. It was concluded that the serum must have contained a 'reagin', a factor which could transfer a specific sensitivity to a single substance.

This elegant experiment remained unexplained, and the presence of 'reagins' remained a theoretical concept for the next 40 years. It was only after the discovery of the immunoglobulins that it was possible for the somewhat nebulous reagins to be identified as immunoglobulin E (IgE) antibodies. These are present in the serum in very small amounts which are, nevertheless, sufficient to attach to and sensitize mast cells which lie below the skin and other body surfaces.

During the years following the experiment of Prausnitz and Küstner, much interest was focused on this remarkable model of 'immunity gone wrong'. Immune reactions, at best, are capable of protecting the body against foreign invaders, whatever their nature. When an immune reaction causes local inflammation, this attracts a variety of scavenger and other inflammatory cells, and a fibrin clot is laid down, thus providing a barrier through which it is difficult for invading organisms or toxic substances to penetrate. As various types of lymphocyte become sensitized, T cells are attracted to the area, thereby adding to the local defence mechanisms.

Antibodies, the products of sensitized B cells, can also display their protective function by circulating to different parts of the body (see Chapter 4). Antibodies of the IgM and IgG class circulate in the bloodstream; IgG, with its different subclasses, also diffuses through the tissues; IgE provides the 'recognition molecules' on the surfaces of inflammation-triggering mast cells; and IgA acts as a coat of 'antiseptic paint' in the mucous secretions. At its best, this combination of events is capable of walling off, destroying, or at least reducing the spread of a large variety of foreign agents which may otherwise be the cause of disease.

Perhaps not surprisingly, exaggerated responses of the body's immune system can itself have unpleasant consequences (Table 5.1). Of the four main types of reaction of which the system is capable, type 1 (immediate allergy) and type 4 (involving T cells) have both been shown to be associated with food allergy. They are considered further as the mechanisms involved in immediate food reactions and coeliac disease respectively.

IMMUNE RESPONSES PROVOKED BY FOOD

Type 1 Reactions

These reactions occur very quickly, usually within minutes – for example, when the IgE-coated mast cells of a food-allergic individual encounter the appropriate food molecules and are triggered into activity (see Chapter 4). Most reactions of this kind are localized, but mast cell

Table 5.1 Types of exaggerated immune response

Type	Mechanism	Examples
1	Immediate allergy (IgE reactions)	Immediate food reactions; hay fever
2	Direct damage by antibody	Blood transfusion reactions[a]
3	Inflammation triggered by immune complexes	Kidney disease (nephritis); 'reactive' arthritis following infections[b]
4	Delayed hypersensitivity (caused by T cells)	Coeliac disease; pneumonitis in food handlers[c]

[a] Also claimed to occur in coeliac disease; unproven
[b] Also suspected in occasional cases of food reactions involving the joints or kidneys; unproven
[c] Unproven

reactions in sensitized individuals have much in common wherever they occur. If a sensitive child develops swelling of the lip or tongue after contact with, for example, egg or nuts, this represents a purely local reaction to contact with the offending substance. Similar reactions can occur in the skin and are, indeed, the basis for the diagnostic tests described in Chapter 6. It has also been shown that, when food solution is applied to the stomach wall through a swallowed tube, reactions will occur in the stomach which are similar to those seen on the mouth or skin (*Reiman et al., 1985*).

Intact food molecules can also be absorbed (see Chapter 4) and diffused throughout the body. As mast cells are present below the skin and below the mucous surfaces of the mouth, intestine and lung airways, absorption of intact food molecules can, in a sensitized subject, lead to a widespread reaction that involves the skin and all mucous linings. A generalized reaction is the exception rather than the rule, however. When it does occur, the result is a generalized anaphylactic response, involving severe symptoms of dramatically sudden onset. The simultaneous release of histamine and other inflammatory agents below the skin and mucosal surfaces throughout the body can result in hives (urticaria), severe asthmatic reactions, local swelling of the skin and underlying tissues (angioedema) and, in the most severe cases, a fall in blood pressure, intestinal colic, coma and even death.

Type 2 Reactions

There is, as yet, no proof that direct damage by antibody is involved in food reactions, although it has been suggested that the IgG antibodies to wheat gliadin found in coeliac disease can cause direct damage to tissues by cross-reacting with a network substance (reticulin) in intestinal cells. The case for believing that wheat gliadin antibodies have a tissue-damaging role is difficult to sustain, however, as the same patients also show IgG antibodies to egg and milk protein unaccompanied by any evidence of clinical sensitivity to those foods. Furthermore, the restriction of gluten in the diet leads to a fall in the level of gliadin antibodies whereas the antibodies to egg and milk persist (Kemeny et al., 1986). This suggests that the antibodies are formed in response to food proteins which cross the mucosal barrier and have little to do with the primary reaction causing the patient's symptoms. IgG antibodies occur in slightly varying forms (subclasses IgG1, 2, 3 and 4), and sensitization to gliadin does not appear to be associated with any of these subclasses.

It has been suggested that an increased permeability of the mucous membrane may be a contributory factor in provoking adverse immunological reactions of various types. When eczema patients with florid food allergy were studied by Barnetson and colleagues (1983), they found that a high proportion had precipitating antibodies to food; they considered this to be evidence suggestive of increased intestinal permeability. More direct tests of permeability have been carried out which measure the extent to which inert molecules of large sugars or edetic acid can penetrate the wall of the intestine and subsequently appear in the urine. By this means, increased permeability has been demonstrated (Walker, 1986) in premature infants, in malnutrition, and in viral gastroenteritis, immunodeficiency, alcoholism (Bjarnason et al., 1984), coeliac disease and a few patients with eczema (Strobel et al., 1984).

Two of the sugars of different molecular size which can be used to measure permeability are cellobiose and mannitol. Using these sugars, Strobel showed that patients with coeliac disease have an increased intestinal permeability to the larger cellobiose molecules not only when they are untreated and have visible damage to their intestinal villi, but also after treatment, when they have apparently normal villi but an excess of lymphocytes – that is, over 40 lymphocytes per 100 villus epithelial cells. Patients with Crohn's disease also showed increased permeability, but this was not an invariable feature of the disease and occurred only when the small bowel was involved.

The evidence thus suggests that diseases associated with an increased permeability of the intestinal mucosa allow the development of an IgG antibody response to food proteins which are able to cross the mucosa, but do not provoke any symptoms or disease. This concept of an increased permeability also applies to patients with clear-cut allergic conditions such as egg allergy, in which other intact food proteins may cross the mucosal membrane. In this condition, IgG antibodies to gliadin are found, presumably reflecting an increased absorption of these molecules across the mucous membrane. There is, however, no clinical evidence of an allergic response to wheat in this condition, which suggests that changes in mucosal permeability do not, by themselves, play a major role in initiating IgE-mediated reactions to food.

Type 3 Reactions

Immune-complex reactions also have a somewhat dubious connection with food reactions. In the absence of any other detectable immune abnormality in some children with cow's milk protein intolerance, the possibility of immune-complex reactions and the activation of complement was, at one time, explored very carefully (*Paganelli et al., 1979; 1981*). Immune complexes containing food can certainly be found in these children, but they also occur in some healthy subjects. The discussion cannot be regarded as closed, however. Immune-complex reactions occur in some types of kidney disease (acute glomerulonephritis) and in a type of arthritis which follows infection. It is therefore worth considering whether the occasional kidney and joint reactions to food (see Chapter 6) could also arise in this way. There is some evidence which supports this view. Immune complexes are usually cleared rapidly from the blood, but a reduced clearance rate has been claimed in one case of food-induced arthritis (*Parke & Hughes, 1981*), and a marginally increased blood level of immune complexes in another (*Panush et al., 1986*).

Type 4 Reactions

In contrast to the uncertainty involved in type 2 and type 3 reactions, type 4 immune reactions, which involve T lymphocytes, can undoubtedly play a part in food intolerance. In a classical study by Marsh (1983), small amounts of gluten were given to coeliac patients who had lost their symptoms while following a gluten-free diet. Samples of their intestinal lining cells were obtained through a swallowed endoscopic tube. Within 12–48 hours, there was a dose-dependent rise in the number of lymphocytes, which were presumed to be in an activated state as there was clear evidence of cell division. On microscopy, there was evidence of the formation of blebs beneath the cells that were associated with separation of the basement membrane. There were also changes that appeared to lead to the activation of mast cells and B cells, and to damage involving the fine, hair-like intestinal villi. As destruction of these villi is the most characteristic feature of coeliac disease, this type of study has provided an opportunity to analyse the step-by-step development of a classical gluten reaction.

A type of lung inflammation seen in food handlers (hypersensitivity pneumonitis) may also represent an example of delayed hypersensitivity due to a type 4 reaction, but this remains unproven (see Chapter 6). It seems possible that, in this condition, immune complexes are also involved.

HOW MUCH IS IMMUNOLOGICAL?

Immediate allergic reactions can be dramatic, but they represent only a minority of all adverse reactions to food. In the oral allergy syndrome, in which the lips, cheeks, tongue or throat may swell or itch within minutes of contact with a specific food, tests for IgE antibodies are nearly always positive. Reactions of a similar type can affect the skin, lungs, or gastrointestinal tract. The foods involved are usually high-protein foods such as eggs, cow's milk, fish and nuts, but reactions can also occur to soya, to spices such as mustard, or to vegetables, for example, celery.

A variety of predisposing factors can also contribute to the clinical response. In individuals who lack secretory IgA, allergic reactions are more likely to occur, but it is not known whether this has an immunological explanation, or whether it reflects the increased susceptibility to intestinal infection and reduced resistance of the mucosal barrier in those who lack the protective action of IgA. Cow's milk protein intolerance can follow closely after a bout of infective gastroenteritis (*Haffejee, 1991*), but the roles of mucosal damage or of infection itself remain uncertain.

Although it is possible that other types of antibody or immune complex can mediate certain food reactions, evidence of an immunological cause is not easy to obtain. Evidence of a cellular immune reaction in coeliac disease has been noted, and a similar mechanism may account for the occasional cases of children who have patchy atrophy of the intestinal villi which appears to be provoked by cow's milk, soya, fish, chicken or rice (*Ament & Rubin, 1972*). There remain, however, many cases in which food-sensitive reactions can be demonstrated by means of challenge tests, but no immunological cause can be identified.

In those reactions in which there is no clear evidence of an immunological cause (*Amlot et al., 1985*), the symptoms range from vomiting and diarrhoea to migraine or other types of headache. While it was, at first, believed that sneezing, a runny nose, asthma, weals on the skin (hives, urticaria), and red weeping rashes (eczema) were always immunological in origin, there is now good evidence that the irritant effect of sulphur dioxide liberated from sulphite preservatives can affect the nose or cause asthma. There is also evidence that urticaria can be provoked by food additives without evidence of any immunological abnormality (*Murdoch et al., 1987*) and that, in some cases, urticaria can be exacerbated by antioxidant food preservatives, and eczema by flavouring agents (see Chapter 7), even when these substances are not the main cause of the reaction (*Goodman et al., 1990*). On current evidence, only a minority of urticaria cases are associated with immunological effects. While eczema usually has an immunological component, that is by no means the whole story. Similarly, intolerance to cow's milk following a bout of gastroenteritis may indicate the development of an allergic reaction, but certainly not in all cases. The clinical syndromes usually regarded to be allergic or food-allergic can also be produced by other mechanisms (Fig. 5.1).

In children, it has long been recognized that irritability and disturbed behaviour can accompany asthma or allergic reactions in other parts of the body. Occasionally, it has been reported that similar behaviour can be observed in children in the absence of any physical

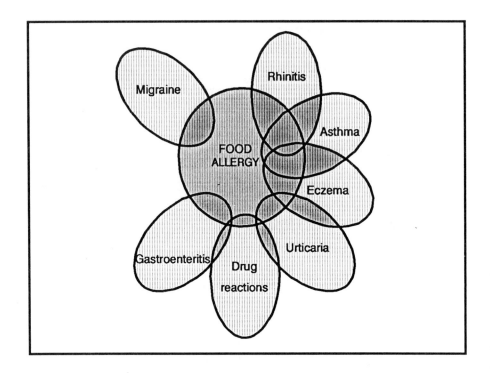

Fig. 5.1

Clinical features that overlap with food intolerance or food allergy. Food allergy can provoke symptoms that are indistinguishable from those of non-allergic forms of rhinitis, asthma, eczema, urticaria, drug reactions, gastroenteritis and migraine. Allergic and non-allergic mechanisms can combine, however, and potentiate one another. In addition, subjects who have been sensitized to food additives (for example, colourings) may show features of a drug reaction which are, in fact, caused by the additives rather than the drug itself.

symptoms. In a large majority of cases, this is easily disproved by challenge tests, but the possibility of occasional mild reactions of this kind has not been entirely excluded (*Pollock & Warner, 1990*).

The wide range of symptoms that can be caused by food include a number of irritable bowel symptoms which are delayed in onset and do not mimic allergic reactions very closely. In other cases, there is a striking clinical resemblance to allergic reactions in the absence of any evidence of a disorder of the immune system. These effects have sometimes been regarded as pseudoallergic, and include toxic and pharmacological effects as well as the consequences of enzyme deficiencies (Table 5.2). However, the clinical pattern is often an

Table 5.2   Main causes of food intolerance

Immunological	Example
Immediate allergy	Swelling in mouth
Other	Coeliac disease
Non-immunological (pseudoallergic)	Example
Toxic	Reactions to fungus-infected food
Drug-like (pharmacological) effects	Caffeinism (and caffeine withdrawal symptoms)
Enzyme defects and digestive deficiencies	Hypolactasia; fat intolerance (various); irritable bowel (some cases)
Multifactorial	Reactions to metabisulphite and other food additives

insufficient basis on which to categorize the type of reaction or to identify the precise cause.

PSEUDOALLERGIC MECHANISMS

Toxic Effects

Naturally occurring toxins are present in a variety of relatively common foods (*Conn, 1973*). These include chemical substances in some potatoes (glycoalkaloids), and in lima beans, millet sprouts and cassava roots (cyanogenic glycosides). In most cases, the toxic effects are only seen when large quantities are eaten (Table 5.3). The toxicity is often lost when the foods are well cooked or, in the case of cassava, when the roots are soaked for long enough to allow the cyanide concentration to fall (*Tylleskar et al., 1992*).

The toxins that arise from fungal or bacterial contamination, or from degenerative changes, can also cause illness in regions where food is poorly stored. As noted in Chapter 4, an example is seen when poorly stored scombroid fish (tuna or mackerel) is kept at temperatures high enough to allow the production of histamine and other biologically active amines which can be toxic at higher concentrations. There are a number of other ways in which toxic effects can be produced by food –

Table 5.3   Foods which can have toxic effects when taken in large quantities

Food	Toxic effect	Prevented by
Lima beans Millet sprouts Cassava roots	Cyanide toxicity (damage to nervous system)	Cooking (or fermentation of cassava)
Cucumbers Beans Berries	Belching Flatus Diarrhoea	Self-limited
Raw red beans	Gastroenteritis	Cooking
Cabbage Turnips Soybeans	Mild goitre	Adequate iodine intake
Liquorice	Sodium retention	Self-limited
Various legumes	Gastroenteritis Red cell agglutination	Cooking

(Derived from *NIH Publication, 1984*)

for example, when repeated reactions to shellfish are caused not by the fish itself, but by the poisonous dinoflagellates on which they have fed.

Not all reactions to food are provoked by oral ingestion. Asthmatics who inhale sulphur dioxide from the metabisulphite in wine or preserved foods can develop asthma within minutes, not through an immunological mechanism, but through a direct irritant effect on the bronchial mucosa. A similar irritant effect may explain sneezing provoked by fizzy drinks. Urticaria and eczema can also develop in the absence of any clear evidence of an IgE reaction.

Pharmacological Effects

Pharmacological food reactions are those which are directly caused by chemicals in foods, of which the best known examples are caffeine and alcohol. The important effects which can be produced by biologically active amines have been discussed in Chapter 4.

The drug-like effects of caffeine are well known. Indeed, caffeine is probably the most common addictive drug in the world. The stimulant effect of 100 mg of caffeine contained in a cup of coffee is so commonplace as to require no further study, and 60 mg of caffeine in a cup of tea can also be an effective stimulant. What is not often realized is that heavy coffee or tea drinkers can suffer the side-effects of caffeine, which stimulates gastric secretion and can cause heartburn, nausea, vomiting and diarrhoea as well as intestinal colic. Irregular heart beats, bouts of rapid pulse, tremor, sweating, sleeplessness and anxiety are also commonplace (*Finn & Cohen, 1978*). Because caffeine is a potent diuretic, it can have a dehydrating effect which may be partly responsible for the irritable bowel symptoms this drug can produce.

The pharmacological effects of alcohol are too well known to require elaboration, but susceptibility to these effects is remarkably variable. It depends especially on the enzyme systems which regulate its metabolism. Some of the problems which may arise are discussed further below.

Pharmacological effects also occur when unusually high quantities of sodium nitrite are ingested. Sodium nitrite is an antioxidant used as a bactericidal agent. In amounts of 20 mg or more, it can dilate the blood vessels, thereby causing flushing and headache, weals on the skin (urticaria) or intestinal symptoms (*Moneret-Vautrin, 1980*).

Enzyme Defects

The most common deficiency of an enzyme known to cause food-intolerant symptoms is hypolactasia, a deficiency of the enzyme lactase that digests milk sugar, lactose. This condition affects up to 80% of the adult population in many parts of the world, a fact which has invited the comment that milk is, after all, a food for babies and not for adults. Lactose levels often fall in later childhood. In patients with hypolactasia, most of the undigested, unabsorbed lactose that reaches the large intestine is fermented by the action of bacteria, which give off hydrogen and carbon dioxide, and produce lactic and propionic acids. The resulting gaseous distention and irritation may be responsible for the many symptoms seen in the irritable bowel syndrome (see Chapter 6), of which cow's milk is a recognized cause (*Levitt et al., 1976*). It remains to be seen how many other cases of food-related intestinal irritability are due to incomplete absorption of food residues and their fermentation in the large bowel.

More than one type of enzyme deficiency can affect the same

metabolic pathway, as in fructose intolerance, which is uncommon but, in its milder forms, may often go undetected. The severe form of aldolase deficiency seen in infants can cause vomiting and rapidly lead to death from liver failure. The condition may be suspected when the urine is tested and found to contain large quantities of amino acids. In fructose diphosphatase deficiency, however, symptoms may only occur intermittently with spells of hyperventilation, hypoglycaemia and ketosis, but the condition is still potentially fatal. In contrast, essential fructosuria due to fructokinase deficiency is a condition which is so benign that it may not attract medical attention and so may not be recognized at all (*Maxwell, 1985*).

Other enzyme deficiencies are now being identified. A deficiency of the enzyme aldehyde dehydrogenase is seen in 40% or more of some Asian communities and is associated with intolerance to alcohol (*Harada et al., 1982*). The symptoms include flushing, breathlessness, a rapid pulse and, after high doses, shock. The effects are similar to those caused by taking alcohol after disulfiram (Antabuse, a drug used in treating alcoholics). Disulfiram interferes with the action of aldehyde dehydrogenase so that, when alcohol is metabolized to acetaldehyde, the metabolic process is arrested at that point and toxic levels of acetaldehyde accumulate. Other drugs, including oral antidiabetic agents, can produce a similar result (*Seixas, 1979*).

As with fructose metabolism, the overall effect is determined by more than one enzyme system, and defects in the metabolism of alcohol can sometimes be overcome. An increased rate of alcohol metabolism can occur at high rates of intake and this has been claimed to be due to a 'microsomal ethanol oxidizing system'. A varying ability to compete with alcohol within this system could explain why some drugs which are prescribed for a variety of medical conditions can have a more potent effect after alcohol, while the effectiveness of other drugs may be completely blocked (*Seixas, 1979*).

As yet, detailed studies have been carried out on only a small number of enzymes which digest or help the absorption or metabolism of food. There may be undiscovered enzyme defects which will help to explain the varying ability of different individuals to tolerate some foods, even in the absence of an immunological explanation. It is becoming more and more apparent that similar clinical manifestations can be produced by more than one mechanism.

Complex Mechanisms

At the clinical level, there is a striking contrast between those patients with food intolerance who react quickly to small quantities of food, and those who react more slowly and can tolerate large and even repeated quantities of a food before symptoms develop. While the second group includes some patients who have mild IgE-mediated reactions – for example, patients who slowly develop eczema, or who have a mild or resolving allergy to cow's milk or eggs – the majority have intestinal reactions for which there is no evidence of an immunological cause. In the case of lactase deficiency (discussed further in Chapter 6), the symptoms are easily explained by the stimulating effect of the gases and acid products released by the fermentation of unabsorbed lactose. Similar symptoms can, however, be produced in other conditions associated with intestinal hurry or the fermentation of unabsorbed food residues. Changes in the character of the bacterial flora inhabiting the lower bowel can also complicate the picture.

When there are unabsorbed food residues, the role of bacterial fermentation in releasing hydrogen is well established (*Levitt et al., 1976*). It has been shown that antibiotics can exacerbate this process by eliminating bacteria which not only produce hydrogen, but also consume it (*Levitt et al., 1974*). This could help to explain why, in some cases, patients with food-provoked irritable bowel symptoms date the onset of their symptoms to an intestinal infection – which could itself play a part – or to the antibiotics given as treatment. Alun Jones (*1985*) has noted that the prophylactic use of metronidazole before gynaecological operations may be followed by food-related irritable bowel symptoms. In pursuing the possibility that the fermentation of unabsorbed food residues could be a factor in these cases, Alun Jones studied affected individuals and carried out bacterial counts in their faeces before and after a specific food challenge. The counts of aerobic bacteria appeared to increase substantially in these circumstances.

CONCLUSION

Food intolerance can no longer be regarded as a single entity. While the most dramatic symptoms are due to anaphylaxis and are nearly always a florid manifestation of IgE-mediated allergic reaction, intolerance to specific foods can also be due to other immunological or non-immunological events. Because different mechanisms are involved, there is no single laboratory test which can identify food intolerance or even provide a broad screening method.

As in other clinical diseases, there is a limit to the ways in which the organ systems of the body can respond to adverse events. Intolerance to a food may be the result of the interplay of different mechanisms and different causes, even when the patient's symptoms are indistinguishable and occur over a similar period of time. The example provided by the simple sugar fructose illustrates that, even when the responsible food is clearly identified, there are occasions when it may be difficult to distinguish between a deficiency of an identifiable enzyme and some other cause.

The diagnostic starting point in all such cases is clinical proof that there is an adverse reaction to food that is reproducible and not influenced by the patient's fears and expectations. Although immediate food reactions are frequently self-diagnosed, an insistence on this diagnosis in the absence of good evidence may reflect an obsessional concern with bodily functions or may mask other features of a depressive illness. It is in such cases – and in children who present with behavioural disorders – that the dangers of misdiagnosis and inappropriate dietary treatment are most in evidence. There is no justification for offering dietary treatment in such cases without valid diagnostic tests and a careful psychiatric assessment.

CHAPTER
—6—

Clinical
Manifestations

ESTABLISHING THE DIAGNOSIS

Validity of Tests

The work of Prausnitz and Küstner (see Chapter 5) showed beyond doubt that, at least in Küstner's case, the serum of an allergic individual contained a substance which reacted specifically with the material which provoked the allergic reaction. This type of specific reaction to a foreign substance is the hallmark of the body's immunological reactions to bacterial and viral infections, and it was then assumed that reactions to food were likely to be immunological in origin. During the next three decades, an increasing number and variety of food reactions were described, including reactions that were often slower and more insidious in onset than Küstner's reaction to fish. Sometimes they involved the gastrointestinal tract and sometimes the skin, or the nose and lungs. In many cases, there was no evidence of an immune response to the food concerned.

In the 1960s, Goldman and co-workers (1963) noted what appeared to be an inverse relationship between the amount of food necessary to provoke a reaction and the rapidity with which the reaction developed. Particularly in children reacting to cow's milk proteins, the slow rate of the development of symptoms in the least sensitive subjects made diagnosis difficult. Goldman therefore emphasized the need to give challenge tests with pure food proteins in a disguised form and to compare the result with the response to inert substances. If necessary, the test could be repeated on several occasions.

The diagnosis of food intolerance is still based on the result of a well conducted food-challenge test but, if there is a history of very severe reactions, the dangers of the test should be considered. There should be personnel and equipment available to treat anaphylactic reactions, should they occur, and small test doses may be helpful. Cow's milk-sensitive infants may require an open challenge with 0.5 ml of milk to be increased or repeated at 30-minute intervals until a skin reaction or respiratory reaction is observed (*Hill et al., 1986*). For the diagnosis of a food allergy rather than other forms of food intolerance, it is also necessary to obtain proof that there is an immunological cause. This is achieved by demonstrating a direct reaction between the food and the patient's skin or serum (Table 6.1).

In differentiating between food intolerance and other disorders, it is necessary to consider a variety of causes of respiratory, gastrointestinal or skin abnormalities. As adverse food reactions are frequently due to non-immunological causes (see Chapter 5), it is important to consider the possibility that an individual's symptoms may be caused by toxins that are present in the food, toxic effects of food contaminants, intestinal or other infective agents, enzyme defects (such as alactasia, which causes cow's milk intolerance), or non-immunological reactions to food additives (such as tartrazine).

Apart from oral challenge tests, the only supplementary diagnostic procedures that have withstood critical examination are a few immunological tests, intestinal biopsy tests, and tests for enzyme deficiences (for example, lactose tolerance tests) or for excessive fermentation in the bowel (as in the breath hydrogen tests; see *Gastrointestinal effects*).

Table 6.1   Clinical diagnosis of food intolerance and allergy

---

- Symptoms should disappear when the food is excluded from the diet.
- Its reintroduction should reproduce the same symptoms even when given in an unrecognizable form.
- The diagnosis of food allergy requires the additional demonstration that the food reacts with cells or antibodies from the patient.

Immunological tests for food sensitivity consist of a limited range of skin tests and a small number of laboratory tests for antibodies to foods. There are very few food extracts suitable for use as skin-test materials but, when appropriate extracts are used, the results of skin-prick tests and intradermal injection tests are surprisingly precise. They depend on the presence of local mast cells which have been sensitized by the attachment of IgE molecules to their surface. When those mast cells are activated by the attachment of food protein to IgE molecules in an individual who has already been sensitized to that food, the mast cells release histamine and other inflammatory substances. The effect of these substances is to make the local capillary walls leak, allowing fluid to diffuse into the tissues, producing a local cutaneous wheal. The high degree of sensitivity and specificity of this type of skin test has been demonstrated in platinum-allergic subjects, who can react to platinum salts at dilutions of 10^{-9} g/ml. Taken together with the amount of solution introduced, this suggests that approximately 100,000 molecules are sufficient to produce a skin wheal.

Although intradermal injections can produce similar results to skin-prick tests, an intradermal injection can itself be traumatic and produce non-specific reactions. The apparent precision of the procedure, therefore, may not be realized in practice. This, together with the expense and the occasional discomfort of the test, has led to its declining popularity in many centres. It remains in vogue among practitioners of alternative medicine, who often inject a variety of substances in many different dilutions. The claims made for such 'titration' procedures have never been validated, however, and the use of a wide range of unstandardized food extracts can give a false impression of scientific accuracy.

The present situation is that only a small number of foods are available in preparations which can provide diagnostic information when used in skin or laboratory tests for food sensitivity. These include the antigenic extracts of egg, white fish, various nuts, and cow's milk. Of these, the least satisfactory are cow's milk preparations, which tend to give negative results even in children with proven cow's milk-protein intolerance. The reason for this is unclear, but a contributory fact is that not all cow's milk reactions are IgE-mediated.

The main laboratory test available for measuring low serum levels of IgE antibody to food is the radioallergosorbent test (RAST). The RAST method can be of considerable value in research procedures or for cross-checking the results of skin-prick tests. It can also be useful in cases in which skin tests will not work because the patient has taken antihistamines or has an overreactive skin. Apart from this, RAST has no intrinsic advantage over the skin-prick test procedure and is often less sensitive.

IgG antibodies to foods are also present in the blood and other body fluids, often as a normal response to small quantities of food proteins which have been absorbed in their natural, undigested form. As noted in Chapter 5, tests for these antibodies are of no diagnostic value.

FOOD INTOLERANCE IN CHILDHOOD

In 1905, Finkelstein reported the death of an infant from an anaphylactic reaction to cow's milk. Since then, a wide variety of symptoms have been attributed to childhood food allergy, and the lively public interest in this subject has sometimes led to alarmist and exaggerated views of both the frequency and the life-threatening nature of reactions of this kind. While allergy may go unrecognized as a cause of a child's illness, the suggestive power of the media is such that there are now many examples of parents who pursue a totally unfounded belief that an apparently healthy child suffers from a food allergy. If clinical tests do not support this diagnosis, it is not uncommon for parents to seek numerous opinions from practitioners of both conventional and alternative medicine until they obtain endorsement for their foregone conclusion. Undoubtedly, there have been instances in which, despite initial medical scepticism, a parent's belief has proved to be well founded on accurate observation. Almost invariably, however, analysis of the more controversial cases has shown psychological and social problems in the family, or has provided clear evidence of an obsessional approach to health that may override all other considerations, and may be accompanied by a refusal to allow any tests to be carried out or to accept the results if they are. In such cases, the use of inappropriate diets may lead to nutritional problems in the child. A form of child abuse is now recognized in which the parent describes fanciful or even fabricated symptoms – the so-called Munchausen's disease by proxy (*Warner, 1984*), named after the imaginative Baron Munchausen of the children's tales.

Incidence

Despite the current trend towards the overdiagnosis of food intolerance, there is no justification for the opposite tendency to minimize the importance of the condition, or to pretend that it does not exist. Food intolerance can cause unpleasant or, in extreme cases, even dangerous symptoms. The most common reaction is to cow's milk, and the estimated incidence of chronic diarrhoea from this cause varies widely – from 0.3–7.5%. As the child's diet broadens, other foods may cause problems, including eggs, fish and soya. In older children and adults, chocolate, peanuts, nuts and berries are not infrequent causes of symptoms. Reactions to cereals are also important, but adverse reactions of the immediate type are relatively uncommon. Reactions to wheat gluten usually present in the form of coeliac disease, wherein the reaction causes damage to the mucous membrane of the small bowel which appears to be associated with a delayed type of hypersensitivity rather than with IgE antibodies. Reactions to wheat can also occur without the other features of coeliac disease and in children with a normal bowel mucosa.

There are still uncertainties as to how sensitization to food first occurs. Reactions to cow's milk protein can be seen in entirely breast-fed infants after their first bottle-feed, and it is presumed that such infants have become sensitized in fetal life, or by cow's milk antigens in breast milk. More commonly, however, the introduction of cow's milk is followed a week or so later by the development of chronic diarrhoea, or an acute gastrointestinal infection is followed by the development of a similar cow's milk-sensitive reaction (*Harrison et al., 1976*), which may be accompanied by evidence of mucosal damage on microscopy (*Kleinman, 1991*). Here again, estimates of prevalence vary in different communities, but it has been claimed that approximately 1.5% of children develop cow's milk-sensitive symptoms according to this pattern.

There is a striking contrast between clinical and laboratory features in children with early and late reactions. Of 100 infants with challenge-proven cow's milk-protein intolerance (*Hill et al., 1986*), 27 reacted within 45 minutes, but there were 17 who reacted more than 20 hours after the start of a challenge procedure which involved the use of cumulative test doses of milk. Positive skin tests were nearly always found in those with immediate reactions to cow's milk, and it is likely that the remainder form a heterogeneous group. Both the early and late type of cow's milk reaction can follow infection but, for example, it is the late reaction that is most likely to develop after a bout of gastroenteritis — at least when rotavirus infection is involved.

When 36 children with well-studied cow's milk intolerance had their serum tested for rotavirus antibodies, 15 had reactions within 40 minutes of a milk challenge, and all except 4 of these had high IgE antibody levels to cow's milk, supporting a diagnosis of allergy. In 10 of these, 15 had negative tests for rotavirus antibodies (*Firer et al., 1988*). There were 21 children, however, who reacted by developing vomiting or diarrhoea 1–24 hours after the milk challenge and who, in contrast to the first group, had negative tests for IgE antibodies to cow's milk, but significantly higher levels of rotavirus antibodies (in 16 of the 21). On the basis of this evidence, it was the non-IgE-mediated reactions which showed a significant association with a previous rotavirus infection.

Rotavirus infections account for up to 89% of hospital admissions for infantile diarrhoea, and about 1 in 5 of the deaths in young children are the result of diarrhoeal diseases. The physiological changes in the intestine are therefore of considerable interest. These involve the invasion by virus and subsequent loss of the absorptive enterocytes, leading to damage to the microvilli and an interference with the absorption of sodium, glucose and water. The areas of damage are patchy, but lactase, maltase and sucrase levels are also depressed (*Haffejee, 1991*). One of the mechanisms leading to clinical problems may therefore be enzyme deficiency. It is on this basis that Hyams (*1981*) recommended a diet which avoids the disaccharide sugars during the postinfective recovery phase in young children.

Haffejee has suggested that, in postinfective cases, the dietary restriction of disaccharide sugars is only necessary in infants who show no improvement after 3–4 days of diarrhoea and are shown to have an excess of reduced sugars in their stool. While this may offer a practical approach to the problem, it leaves a number of unanswered questions concerning the relationship between postinfective intestinal damage and either a transient food intolerance or a more prolonged process of sensitization, which may affect the baby's tolerance of cow's milk over a longer period.

In developing countries, the position is further complicated by the fact that many children, whether well or poorly nourished, have large numbers of bacteria in the upper part of the small bowel. This, in turn, leads to a high concentration of free bile acids in the bowel lumen that interferes with both the normal digestion of fatty acids by lipase and the mixing of bile with fatty acids, which is a prelude to their absorption. There is therefore − even in apparently healthy children − some impairment of absorption of fat and fat-soluble substances. In some cases, bacterial colonization also contributes to the partial villous atrophy of the jejunum and ileum that is a not uncommon finding in some areas (*Iyngkaran et al., 1979*).

It has also been suggested that acute intestinal infection can lay the basis for a subsequent sensitivity reaction to milk or soy (*Walker Smith, 1982; Iyngkaran et al., 1988*). Small intestinal mucosal damage (enteropathy) can certainly occur in children with intestinal reactions to a number of foods (*Iyngkaran et al., 1978*) and is not confined to coeliac disease (see Chapter 9). Serial biopsies of the small intestine, before and after dietary exclusion and food challenge, have shown that food-induced small intestinal mucosal damage also occurs in children with sensitivity to cow's milk protein, egg, soya, gluten, rice, chicken and fish (*Vitoria et al., 1982; Iyngkaran et al., 1982*). In cow's milk-sensitive enteropathy, the mucous membrane damage is variable in severity. The mucosa is thin, the numbers of intraepithelial lymphocytes are increased, and there is an accumulation of fat in the epithelium. These changes are rapidly reversed when cow's milk is withdrawn from the diet (*Walker Smith, 1986*).

The diagnosis of cow's milk intolerance is based on the history of symptoms and sometimes supported by laboratory tests but, as in other types of food intolerance, the results of oral challenge can be conclusive. Those whose symptoms clear when cow's milk is avoided and return when it is reintroduced are assumed to be cow's milk-intolerant. Children with a family history of allergy and a raised total level of IgE in the cord blood at birth (> 0.5 μ/ml) are more likely to develop cow's milk-protein intolerance as well as other allergic problems. Indeed, infants with early IgE sensitization to cow's milk have been reported to have a 38% chance of developing adverse reactions to other foods (especially egg) before the age of 3 years, and a 48% chance of developing allergic rhinitis or asthma (*Host & Halken, 1990*).

Skin-prick tests with cow's milk or milk protein can help to confirm the diagnosis if the results are positive, but are usually unhelpful. Although blood tests for IgG antibodies to milk proteins can be carried out, their presence both in normal and atopic individuals makes them useless for diagnostic purposes (*Kemeny et al., 1991*).

In the cow's milk-intolerant infant, vomiting, abdominal pain and diarrhoea can occur; there may be other symptoms (Table 6.2), including angioedema, wheezing or even acute anaphylaxis, which may be sufficiently severe to require adrenaline, corticosteroids, intravenous fluids and other resuscitative measures, and may even result in death if left untreated. There have also been cases of infantile colitis, in which persistent bloody diarrhoea and a superficial ulceration of the lower bowel has subsided when cow's milk feeds have been replaced by soya milk (*Jenkins et al., 1984*). A syndrome of blood-streaked, soft stools has also been described in which only the rectum is involved (benign proctitis) and subsides when breast-feeding is stopped and casein hydrolysates given instead (*Lake, 1991*). In most cases, sensitization has been shown to have occurred to a single food in the mother's diet. When that food is eliminated, breast-feeding has again been possible

Table 6.2   Clinical manifestations of cow's milk allergy

- Gastrointestinal
    Vomiting
    Colic
    Diarrhoea
    Intestinal obstruction

- Respiratory
    Rhinitis
    Asthma
    Recurrent cough

- Dermatological
    Angioedema
    Urticaria
    Eczema

- Nervous system
    Irritability
    Convulsions
    Sleep disturbances
    Headache

- Other
    Anaphylaxis
    Iron deficiency anaemia (due to intestinal bleeding)

---

without incident. Occasionally, children with cow's milk sensitivity can also develop a chronic form of lung disease accompanied by the deposition of iron in the tissues (pulmonary haemosiderosis; *Bahna & Heiner, 1980*). More common than these and second only to milk-induced diarrhoea in its frequency is the development of eczema. The clinical features of this condition are discussed below.

Infantile Eczema

A family history of allergic disorders is most commonly found in children with eczema, most of whom have positive, immediate skin reactions to dust mites or foods; 20% also develop asthma and 45% have hay fever (*Price, 1987*). The condition has become much more frequent, possibly doubling or trebling in incidence in the years since World War II (*Wadsworth, 1985*).

Three-quarters of all cases of childhood eczema develop in the first year of life. Itching is often intense and patches of redness, whether on the cheeks or elsewhere, tend to be rubbed and scratched until they develop into a weeping, crusted and often infected rash of the face, scalp, and the more accessible surfaces of the limbs and trunk. Adverse reactions to foods are often important. In a controlled study, around 50% of a selected group of eczematous children developed a red rash after double-blind food challenges (*Sampson, 1983*). When milk, wheat or eggs are involved, intestinal symptoms are often associated, and the first rash to develop may be urticarial, followed by a diffuse flushing and the typical changes of eczema. The condition tends to improve or disappear by the age of 5 years but, when it persists, the folds of skin in front of the elbows or behind the knee are most frequently affected together with the hands, face and scalp.

In addition to attempts to identify and exclude any food that may be contributory to the problem, the treatment of eczema consists essentially of the avoidance of woollen clothing, the use of aqueous creams or oatmeal preparations rather than ordinary soap, and the use of emulsifying ointments after a bath to help keep the skin moist. Further details of treatment are given by Price (*1987*).

Preventive measures
As eczema is so much more common in families with a history of allergy, it should be possible to apply preventive measures in babies identified as being at risk. Although strenuous efforts have been made

to develop appropriate protocols for the diet of both mother and baby, no regime has been sufficiently reliable in preventing this skin condition. A reasonable case has been made for the avoidance of large quantities of milk or eggs in the diet of the mother during the last 3 months of pregnancy. Several controlled studies have also shown that exclusive breast-feeding for the first 3 months of life can substantially reduce the incidence of eczema in the infant, and there is enough evidence to justify a policy of deferring the introduction of eggs, fish and solid food for a further 2–3 months. In any given individual, none of these measures can guarantee that eczema will not develop either while these dietary measures are followed or after they have been stopped.

The suggestion that soya proteins may provide a useful substitute for cow's milk in children who are at risk has not proved successful in practice. Soya proteins appear to be at least as antigenic as cow's milk proteins, and the sugar content of various commercial preparations can also influence the outcome. Those containing sucrose tend to be associated with diarrhoea (*Donovan & Torres-Pinedo, 1987*).

One advance that has been made in the prevention of cow's milk-protein intolerance has been the introduction of feeds based on casein hydrolysates, in which the milk protein has been broken down to smaller molecules. These hydrolysates appear to be better tolerated than cow's milk itself in children who have had recent cow's milk-intolerant symptoms. Although they may be useful – especially when reintroducing milk preparations after a period of illness – hydrolysates have a distinctly unpleasant taste and tend to be expensive.

Childhood Asthma

The prevalence of asthma varies widely in different parts of the world. Around 11% of primary school children in Newcastle, England were found to have recurrent episodes of wheezing (*Lee et al., 1983*). While comparisons may be difficult because of the different diagnostic criteria used in different surveys, there has been, over the past 40 years, a steady increase in the reported prevalence of asthma in children. This cannot be explained solely in terms of a greater awareness among doctors or a greater willingness to make the diagnosis. During the past 15 years, a period during which diagnostic criteria have not changed, the number of children admitted to hospital with asthma has increased steadily, with nearly twice as many admissions during the months of summer and autumn as during those of winter and spring. Thirty per cent of asthmatic children miss more than 3 weeks of schooling each year.

Some of the factors that trigger asthmatic attacks are listed in Table 6.3. Although it is unusual for an asthmatic child to identify foods as precipitating attacks of coughing or wheezing, a survey of children attending a hospital asthma clinic showed that three-quarters of them were able to recall attacks of wheezing provoked by at least one article of food (*Wilson, 1984*). In addition to milk, egg, fish and nuts, which are the most common foods, iced and fizzy drinks (particularly cola) were frequently cited, and it was noted that food- or drink-induced asthma was more common in Asian children than in other ethnic groups. In spite of these clear accounts, these observations often cannot be confirmed by double-blind challenge tests in laboratory conditions. Wilson's further work has shown, however, that challenge tests which do not cause an asthmatic attack may nevertheless increase the sensitivity of the bronchial airways to the point where any additional stimulus, such as the inhalation of histamine 30 minutes after a food challenge, can provoke an asthmatic attack much more readily than previously (*Wilson & Silverman, 1985*). The duration of this phenomenon may be short-lived. When methacholine inhalations were given 24 hours after a food challenge, Zuretchkenbaum and colleagues (*1991*) were unable to demonstrate a significant effect.

It is certainly not a new suggestion that agents which provoke asthma may complement one another. Trousseau was a distinguished, but somewhat bad-tempered, French physician of the nineteenth century who was himself an asthmatic. He observed that, when he was under emotional stress, an asthmatic episode could be exacerbated, but he also noticed that the attack itself was provoked by close contact with

Table 6.3 Factors which provoke wheezing attacks in asthmatic children

Throat and chest infections
Allergy (dust mites, pollen, pets, food)
Non-allergic food reactions (e.g. sulphites in food)
Other irritants (e.g. smog, cigarette smoke)
Emotion
Gastric reflux

horses. If he quarrelled with his coachman while in the stable, he would invariably suffer an asthmatic attack. Going into the stable alone, or quarrelling with the coachman out in the open, had no such effect. The same principle may apply to other situations. In asthmatic children, as in adults, the additive effect of food and other factors can be striking. It should be noted, however, that food intolerance is more likely to potentiate asthma than to cause it. Food which can provoke an asthmatic attack when the affected person is frightened or takes exercise may have no effect in relaxed surroundings. When there is a history of asthmatic reactions which have been provoked by a food on several occasions, the fact that the food can sometimes be taken with impunity, or may not always cause asthma during a challenge test, does not necessarily mean that the original observation was wrong. In such cases, a challenge test should be repeated, or followed by exercise, before accepting a negative result.

Other Childhood Symptoms

Headache and other neurological symptoms, joint pains, and reactions involving the kidney and blood platelets are considered later in this chapter. Sneezing and nasal obstruction have also been well described and may persist, leading to the diagnosis of 'chronic rhinitis'. This is usually seen in conjunction with other symptoms (*Atkins et al., 1985*; *Pastorello et al., 1985*; *Pelikan & Pelikan-Filpek, 1987*). Among these are deafness due to serous otitis media which, despite much controversy, has been shown to occur during double-blind food challenges (*Friedman et al., 1983*).

REACTIONS IN OLDER CHILDREN AND ADULTS

The normal infant's response to a newly encountered food antigen is that of tolerance. When tolerance has developed, repeated encounters with the same antigen will elicit a similar, tolerant response. In contrast – partly through the discriminating effect of the Peyer's lymphoid patches – bacteria and bacterial antigens provoke an immune reaction which can eliminate the foreign matter and provide a capacity to produce antibodies that will reject similar material briskly on subsequent occasions. The development of allergy to food instead of tolerance can therefore be regarded as a failure of the normal tolerizing mechanism. The part played by genetic factors or by intestinal infection in this 'breaking of tolerance' is still not fully understood, and the duration of the adverse effect is variable.

Immediate allergic reactions of the IgE type differ from other antibody reactions of infancy and show a greater tendency to disappear spontaneously. When an infant develops an immune-complex-mediated hypersensitive response to a food such as cow's milk, it may not persist for more than a few months, and children who are even older may lose their sensitivity with time. Bock (1985) has estimated that 40% of food-intolerant children below the age of 3 years will have lost their food sensitivity within 1–2 years. A remission rate of 19% was noted in children over this age. Remission rates vary, however, with the type of food involved. The majority of children with cow's milk-protein intolerance lose their sensitivity as they become older. In contrast, those who are sensitive to peanuts are not only prone to severe reactions (*Moneret-Vautrin et al., 1991*), but seldom become tolerant in later life (*Bock & Atkins, 1989*). The more insidious type of food sensitivity represented by coeliac disease (see Chapter 9) is nearly always a lifelong problem, although its severity may diminish.

In the adult, as in the child, there are problems both in explaining and in diagnosing the onset of an adverse reaction to food in a previously tolerant subject. Food reactions have been blamed for a wide range of symptoms, not all of which can be reproduced by means of challenge tests. In making a diagnosis, the need to consider food fads and psychiatric illness has already been discussed. Patients with a wide range of gastrointestinal diseases may also notice unpleasant food-related symptoms, often provoked by a particular class of substances, such as fats, rather than a specific food. Such a history by itself is of limited value unless the reaction is reproducible on challenge and in the absence of any evidence of underlying disease of another type.

Food Antigens and Cross-Reactions

The most common foods causing specific food-intolerant reactions are listed in Table 6.4. The frequency of reactions to different foods varies with the types of diet in different parts of the world, which should therefore be taken into account. Some of the foods that provoke different immunological reactions are also capable of causing food

Table 6.4 Foods most frequently causing symptoms of food intolerance

Commonly involved foods

Milk[a]	Nuts, peanuts[a]	Rice[b]
Egg[a]	Pork, tenderized meat,	Chick peas[b]
Wheat, cereals, yeast	papain	Coffee, tea
Fish[a], shellfish[a]	Chocolate	Preservatives
	Citrus fruit	Other additives

Other foods reported to cause reactions

Aniseed	Clove	Peas
Apple[a]	Fennel	Peach, other soft fruit
Artichoke	Garlic, onion	Peppers (various)
Banana	Ginger	Potato
Beans (various)	Herbs (e.g. bay leaf)	Sesame[a]
Beetroot	Honey	Seeds (various)
Berries (various)	Hops	Soya[a]
Camomile	Horseradish	Sweet potato
Celery[a]	Mango	Tapioca
Chestnut	Millet	Vanilla
Chicken	Mushroom	
Chicory	Mustard[a]	
Cinnamon	Nutmeg	

[a] Often involving the immediate type of reaction
[b] In Asian countries, but not in the West, where reactions to these foods are uncommon.
(*Niphadkar et al., 1992*)

intolerance in other ways. Cow's milk reactions, for example, can be IgE-mediated, but cow's milk can also affect people who cannot tolerate lactose because they lack the enzyme lactase. Gluten intolerance occurs in patients with coeliac disease, but Cooper and co-workers (*1980*) have shown that gluten-sensitive diarrhoea can occur in non-coeliac patients; IgE-mediated reactions to wheat have also been reported (*Dohi et al., 1991*). To complicate matters further, there are also patients who appear to react only to white flour or to processed wheat products.

Cross-sensitization provides a further diagnostic problem presumably because of the molecular similarity between proteins of similar biological origin. Patients who present with hay fever provoked by silver birch tree pollen are often allergic to the soft fruit of several other trees (*Halmepuro & Bjorksten, 1985*), or to manufactured food products containing soya flour as a minor ingredient. Allergy to latex rubber (another tree product) can be closely associated with allergy to fruit, especially bananas and chestnuts (*Lavaud et al., 1992; Ceuppens et al., 1992*). Patients who are allergic to birch or mugwort pollen can also react to celery (*Wattrich et al., 1990*), and ragweed allergy is sometimes associated with sensitivity to melon and banana (*Andersson et al., 1970*). Furthermore, patients who are sensitive to soya can react to botanically related legumes, such as peas, beans and lentils (*Fries, 1971*). They may also encounter difficulties not because of cross-reactions, but because soy has been so frequently incorporated into processed food products that cereal mixtures, soups, sauces, biscuits, baked foods, and infant formula feeds may all contain soy.

As a practical point, those who are sensitive to soya protein may be able to take the commercial soya oils which are added to margarine (*Bush et al., 1985*). This may depend on the purity of the oil, as a similar claim has been made (*Taylor et al., 1981*) that peanut oil does not affect peanut-sensitive individuals, although this is not always so (see Chapter 8, pages 147–8).

Cross-reactions are also in evidence in the tests which are used in diagnosis. Radioallergosorbent (RAST) tests carried out on patients with hay fever frequently give positive results with wheat flour (*Lessof et al., 1980*), so it may be difficult to distinguish the test results of these patients from those with immediate reactions to wheat, even those with florid skin reactions, oedema, asthma, or rhinitis (*Walsh et al., 1987*). Although the use of more refined flour extracts has been claimed to solve this problem, more evidence is needed that they can discriminate between wheat-intolerant subjects and those hay-fever sufferers who have IgE antibodies to grasses which cross-react with cereal proteins (*Donovan & Baldo, 1990*) but who have no difficulty in eating cereal foods.

Clinical Features

In the most severe cases, such features as vomiting and anaphylactic shock can develop within minutes, together with asthma, a fall in blood pressure, and extensive urticaria. The quantity of food needed to trigger the attack can be very small. In highly sensitive infants, an attack can be provoked by less than 1 ml of milk (*Savilahti, 1981*) and, in older children or adults, by small fragments of nut concealed in a mouthful of cake. Even the contamination of restaurant utensils or the food manufacturing plant (*Gern et al., 1990*) can occasionally cause severe reactions. A variety of other symptoms occur (Fig. 6.1), including abdominal pain, bloating and constipation.

The development of a reaction within minutes of eating a food has often been taken as presumptive evidence of an IgE-mediated reaction. This is almost always true in individuals who develop swelling of the lips or tongue, blebs of local swelling inside the mouth or tightness of the throat (*Amlot et al., 1985*). When the presenting symptom is asthma, however, this may not be the case, as inhaled sulphur dioxide can provoke asthma by a direct toxic effect on the mucous lining of the bronchi (see Chapter 5).

In anaphylaxis, as in asthma, immunological and non-immunological events can potentiate the response to food. Food-dependent exercise-induced anaphylaxis has been reported by many observers since Maulitz and colleagues (*1979*) first recounted the case history of the long-distance runner who had strongly positive tests for IgE antibodies to

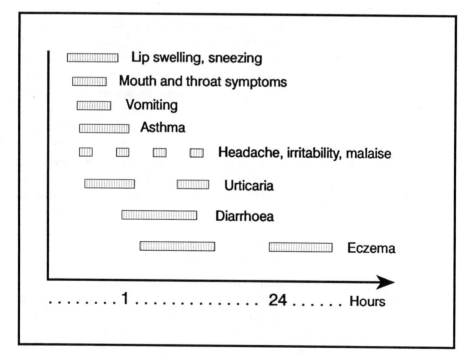

Fig. 6.1
Food intolerance: Time course of the appearance of symptoms.

shellfish. He could eat shellfish with impunity or run for long distances without any side-effects. He developed a severe anaphylactic reaction, however, if he ate shellfish several hours before going for a run. More recently, Dohi and colleagues (*1991*) studied 11 patients who all had recurrent episodes of anaphylaxis when exercise was taken after food. They found that only in seven cases were these associated with a specific food (shellfish, wheat or grape), and all had correspondingly positive skin-prick tests. The remaining four could not identify any specific food, but the act of eating appeared to predispose to anaphylaxis. When other potentiating factors were sought, two reported that their most severe attacks occurred when they had also taken aspirin. Fatigue, cold and lack of sleep were suspected of having an exacerbating effect. Beta-blocking drugs have also been thought to make anaphylaxis worse (*Hannaway & Hopper, 1983*) and to reduce the effect of adrenaline in treatment. Patients who have a history of anaphylactic reactions should therefore alert their physicians if they need prescriptions for other conditions – for example, for hypertension. A Medicalert bracelet may help to ensure that the patient's problem is not forgotten or overlooked.

It has already been noted that delayed reactions that only occur after substantial quantities of food are taken are seldom immunological. In many cases, the specificity of the reaction is difficult to establish. The differential diagnosis includes not only lactose intolerance and other enzyme deficiencies, but also peptic ulceration and gallstones, cystic fibrosis, other conditions associated with fatty diarrhoea, low-grade intestinal infections, the pharmacological effects of caffeine, and psychological illness.

Gastrointestinal effects

The symptoms of food intolerance include vomiting, diarrhoea, abdominal pain and distention, constipation, and a variety of symptoms due to fat malabsorption or, in unusual cases, to protein loss into the bowel. Itching of the anus is not uncommon in patients with diarrhoea, and there may be inflammatory changes in the rectum and even bleeding in association with cow's milk intolerance (*Buisseret et al., 1978*).

The symptoms observed in these gastrointestinal patients are summarized in Table 6.5. Recurrent minor episodes of bleeding can lead to an iron-deficiency anaemia, and low serum-protein levels may be found usually in severely ill patients who also have other problems,

Table 6.5 Gastrointestinal reactions to food

- Direct effects
  Vomiting, diarrhoea, pain, bloating, constipation
- Secondary effects
  Fatty diarrhoea, blood loss and iron deficiency, loss of protein, eosinophilic gastroenteritis
- Remote effects
  Runny nose, asthma, urticaria, angioedema, eczema, anaphylaxis

such as asthma and eczema. Fatty diarrhoea due to cow's milk intolerance is probably more common than has been realized; Kuitunen and colleagues (1975) were able to describe 54 such cases. Fatty diarrhoea is, nevertheless, not a common feature of food allergy, and is most often seen in gluten-sensitive patients who have coeliac disease.

The more dramatic and immediate gastrointestinal reactions present a relatively simple diagnostic problem in which the triggering agent is often easily identified. There may be accompanying allergic features outside of the intestinal tract. It is, in general, the more insidious reactions that are most difficult to identify and, in such cases, it is important to consider the non-immunological causes described in Chapter 5, including toxic and pharmacological effects.

Reactions which develop hours, days or weeks after the first introduction of a food may nevertheless be severe, as in the children described earlier (see pages 93–4) who have intestinal mucosal damage. Except in coeliac disease, such changes are not seen in adults, but adults may nevertheless describe a similar, cumulative development of symptoms or an apparently incongruous response – for example, hypolactasia in which the tolerance of cow's milk may vary from one day to the next, or symptoms of the irritable bowel syndrome that may be almost indistinguishable from those caused by other conditions associated with diarrhoea or malabsorption. Confusion may also arise when individuals who cannot tolerate the lactose in cow's milk can nevertheless enjoy yoghurt, which contains lactase-producing bacteria.

Secondary lactase deficiency can also arise, particularly when giardiasis, coeliac disease or severe infectious diarrhoea damages the enterocyte brush border or denudes the intestinal mucosa (*Burke et al., 1965; Iyngkaran et al., 1979*). A lactose tolerance test or a lactose breath-hydrogen test can then help to identify the cause, as hydrogen and other gases resulting from the fermentation of unabsorbed lactose are absorbed into the bloodstream. On reaching the lungs, they are easily detected when they are exhaled in the expired air.

A further problem was identified by Alun Jones and colleagues (1982), who investigated patients who had no evidence of alactasia or intestinal disease but, nevertheless, complained of nausea, bloating, abdominal pain and either constipation or, more usually, diarrhoea. It transpired that many of these patients showed an increase in symptoms when given the treatment which was then in vogue – a high-residue diet with a high bran content. Their symptoms tended to improve when a more limited diet was prescribed. A double-blind study was then carried out in which these patients were challenged with either flavoured pureed food preparations or similarly flavoured 'control' mixtures. Two-thirds of the patients developed gastrointestinal symptoms after taking specific foods, sometimes accompanied by objective evidence of an increased release of prostaglandins in the rectum. The foods most commonly involved were wheat and other cereal foods, but milk products, coffee and tea, eggs, citrus fruits and a variety of vegetables also provoked symptoms in some patients. Nanda and his colleagues (1989) have noted that chocolate, onions, nuts, potato and alcohol can cause problems in some individuals.

In contrast to the irritable bowel syndrome, in which there are changes in bowel function but no structural changes, intestinal reactions to food may occasionally be associated with other detectable abnormalities, for example, a high level of eosinophilic white cells in the peripheral blood. Some of the patients with eosinophilia also have a diffuse infiltration in the wall of the stomach or intestinal tract, usually with symptoms suggesting an allergic reaction elsewhere in the body, ranging from nasal symptoms to angioedema, urticaria and asthma (Klein et al., 1970). This is called eosinophilic gastroenteritis, a condition that can range from mild to severe, or even be fatal. A number of specific reactions to foods have been reported in eosinophilic gastroenteritis (Nelson et al., 1979). A recent case report (Mazza et al., 1991) has drawn attention to the fact that it can occur in acquired immunodeficiency syndrome (AIDS), when a rising IgE level may reflect the disordered IgE antibody regulation that can occur with the loss of T-lymphocyte control mechanisms. In Mazza's patient, vanilla ice cream and tangerines caused symptoms of both gastroenteritis and of angioedema.

In eosinophilic gastroenteritis, dietary restriction (*Caldwell et al.*, *1975*) often does not reverse all of the features of the disease. The addition of corticosteroids may be necessary for control of symptoms.

In contrast to the association of infantile colitis with cow's milk-protein intolerance, there is no evidence that food allergy plays any part in the very different condition of ulcerative colitis in adults. Although an association was, at one time, suspected because the exclusion of cow's milk was sometimes of benefit, this effect and the presence of IgG antibodies to cow's milk proteins appear to be the secondary consequence of mucosal damage. Crohn's disease of the bowel may also benefit from dietary restriction but, again, the available evidence suggests that this is a secondary effect.

Skin reactions

Skin reactions to food are common in childhood, and the parent who observes a widespread, red 'strawberry' rash or a bright red flush around the lips when a child takes an orange drink is unlikely to consult a doctor. More troublesome rashes can occur, such as urticarial reactions to cow's milk or hen's egg, and sensitization of the intact skin may occur in children who develop contact urticaria after merely touching egg or fish. The urticaria in food-allergic patients is usually brief, lasting only a few hours. Characteristically, the presence of immediate sensitivity can be confirmed in such cases by skin-prick tests.

There is a limit to the number of ways in which the skin can react, and urticaria has a number of different causes. Provocation by food accounts for only a minority of cases (Table 6.6). In the aftermath of an attack, recurrences may sometimes be provoked by non-specific factors, such as warmth, exercise, and possibly foods with a high amine

Table 6.6 Classification of urticaria

---

1. Caused by histamine-containing or -releasing food
2. Caused by immunological reaction to foods, drugs, parasites or injected substances (including venoms)
3. Physical urticaria (e.g. provoked by cold, pressure, sunshine)
4. Urticaria associated with inflammatory diseases involving blood vessels (e.g. systemic lupus)
5. Hereditary angioedema
6. Chronic urticaria of unknown origin

---

content. The reason for this liability to recurrences is not clear, although it has been suggested that it may involve a depletion or change in activity of the enzymes diamine oxidase and methyltransferase. As these enzymes are responsible for the inactivation of histamine, their depletion could enhance the activity of any histamine absorbed by food or released from mast cells. It has been argued that, as mast cell activation triggers a discharge of diamine oxidase from the intestinal mucosal cells and leaves them depleted, this may result in a temporarily increased susceptibility to recurrences of urticaria, triggered by the effects of toxic diamines of dietary and bacterial orgin (*Lessof et al., 1990*). Furthermore, there may be other circumstances in which the activity of diamine oxidase is diminished, for example, by alcohol (*Sessa et al., 1984*). Less is known, however, of the factors that influence the activity of methyltransferase.

Eczema in adults

Eczema in early childhood has already been discussed. In older subjects, eczema is an itchy red rash often involving the skin creases as well as the hands, face and other regions where the secondary effects of scratching and bacterial infection may supervene. The lesions are prone to blistering, scaling and, in many cases, exudation of fluid and crusting. An association with allergy is very commonly seen, especially in cases of early onset. In addition to the associated presence of asthma, allergic nasal problems, and a family history of allergy, a high serum IgE level frequently provides further support for an allergic origin. However, the slow evolution of the skin reaction and the dense infiltration of lymphocytes on microscopy are more suggestive of delayed hypersensitivity than of the immediate-type allergic response. This may, in part, be due to the changes which supervene when acute reactions are provoked repeatedly on several occasions, and gradually change in nature.

It has already been noted that food allergy is a very potent provoking factor in childhood eczema, but the rash may have urticarial features at the onset. Meara (*1965*) was able to study 29 children who had both atopic eczema and a positive skin-prick test to egg. On an egg-free diet, 11 of these children improved but, when egg was reintroduced, eight responded by developing urticaria and only two developed eczema. The initial acute reaction was clearly different from that which developed at a later stage. Similar observations have been made in the even more common cases of eczema in association with cow's milk-protein intolerance.

Asthma in adults

About one in every six asthmatic patients believe that particular foods can provoke an asthmatic attack (Burr, 1980). In some, inhaled odours can provoke an attack, and the smell of fish may be sufficient to induce asthma in fish-allergic individuals. There are other cases in which the ingestion of food may be followed by an asthmatic attack 1–2 hours later (Papageorgiou et al., 1983), in which case, it is less likely that the inhalation route is involved. The route by which foods can trigger an asthmatic attack can thus vary from one patient to another.

There are also differences between the mechanisms involved in food-provoked asthmatic episodes. These include the irritant effects of sulphur dioxide, the immediate IgE-mediated allergy associated with fish odours, and the delayed response reported in the case of milk, which may be unassociated with any evidence of an IgE response (Lessof et al., 1980). There are also variations in the way individuals react to the various components of a single food; for example (Gershwin et al., 1985), four out of 24 asthmatics had an asthmatic episode after drinking a glass of white wine, as indicated by a sharp reduction in the volume of air they were able to breathe out in 1 second (FEV_1). Subsequent studies with flavoured drinks showed that sodium metabisulphite in an alcohol-free mixture could provoke asthma in one case, but this had no effect in another subject who nevertheless developed asthma after drinking alcohol itself.

Other lung conditions have occasionally been suspected in food-sensitive subjects; for example, patients with coeliac disease and an abnormal intestinal mucosa may absorb intact food proteins through their damaged intestinal wall and become sensitized to hen's egg (Faux et al., 1978). It has been suggested that this may explain the tendency to develop a type of lung reaction known as 'bird-fancier's lung', a condition seen in individuals who have close contact with birds, or who clean the cages of pigeons and thus inhale dried bird proteins, thereby stimulating a further immune response (Berrill et al., 1975).

Diagnosis of Food-Induced Asthma

When an asthmatic response to food is suspected, the patient should take home a peak flow meter and keep a record of breathing capacity over a period of days or weeks, correlated with a diary of the food intake

(*Wraith, 1980*). At its simplest, this may reveal a consistent drop in peak flow value after the intake of a particular food. More difficult to analyse are those insidious and prolonged episodes of bronchospasm which follow more than one food and may be influenced, in addition, by precipitating factors such as exercise, cold weather, or contact with animal proteins and dust mites. The additive effects of different provoking factors can be striking, especially when exercise and an allergic reaction are combined (*Maulitz et al., 1979*), or when an acute asthmatic attack is provoked sufficiently often to lead to cell infiltration and inflammation and, thus, change its nature. It is clear that the time course of food-related asthma can be short after a single episode but, as in eczema, there may be an insidious change in the type of asthma that develops after repeated challenge with a particular food. In such cases, reversible spasm of the bronchial smooth muscle is no longer the main component. The long time-scale may then be reminiscent of that seen in occupational asthma, where the immediate relationship to exposure becomes blurred because of the repeated inhalation of industrial chemicals. The remission which at first occurs on leaving work may then take longer and longer to achieve, as demonstrated by the patient's own breathing pattern, recorded with the help of a peak flow meter. As in occupational asthma, the onset of the asthmatic episodes provoked by food can follow a slow time-scale and after repeated exposure, the remission which follows food withdrawal may be equally slow.

Headache, Migraine and Neurological Symptoms

Hippocrates noted that '. . . milk is not recommended for those who suffer from headaches . . .' and that '. . . sweet wine is less likely to produce headache than is heavy wine . . .' More recently, food has been recognized as one of the agents which can provoke migraine, and there have been numerous reports of the triggering effect of alcohol, dairy products (including cheese), chocolate, fish, eggs, nuts and beans (*Hanington, 1983; Mansfield et al., 1985; Vaughan & Mansfield, 1991*).

Migraine is a headache that recurs at intervals. It is usually felt mainly on one side of the head, and is frequently associated with nausea and sometimes vomiting. In about half of those affected, these symptoms are preceded or accompanied by flashing lights or other eye symptoms, and occasionally by sensory and speech disturbances or even migrainous hemiplegia. Approximately 8% of the general population suffer from this condition. It is rare in early childhood, but becomes more common later, especially in women during the child-bearing years, one in five of whom may be affected at one time or another. There is a strong family incidence. Two-thirds of migraine sufferers can identify a parent, brother, sister or grandparent who have also suffered in this way.

During a migraine attack, there is evidence of depressed function of the brain, starting posteriorly and spreading forwards steadily at about 2–3 mm/min (*Lauritzen & Olesen, 1987*). The triggering event, however, appears to involve changes in the degree of distention of the cerebral blood vessels, which occur both before and during the headache phase. A reversible dilatation of the large intracranial arteries can be demonstrated (*Friberg et al., 1991*), and one of the most effective anti-migraine drugs, sumatriptan, appears to abolish this dilatation, especially in the small linking blood vessels (anastomoses) between arteries and veins (*Anon, 1992*).

Migraine can be influenced by a number of factors which act on blood vessels, including those which increase the absorption of biologically active amines or their release within the body (*Hanington & Lessof, 1987*). In particular, 5-hydroxytryptamine (serotonin) has been shown to play an important part. This substance is present in a number of foods, is stored and released by blood platelets, and causes blood vessel constriction in a variety of tissues, where it acts upon three different types of cell receptor. By binding to the first of these receptors, sumatriptan interposes itself in the serotonin pathway, and this may be the basis of its anti-migraine activity.

The potential effect of food upon these complex mechanisms is small. Biologically active amines are released during physical and mental stress, and fatigue, excitement and anger are prominent among the precipitating factors which can have a cumulative effect in triggering a migraine attack (see Fig. 6.2). Once an attack has occurred, there is usually a refractory period before another can begin, but it is not known whether this is because the platelets have lost their serotonin stores.

Fig. 6.2
Vascular factors in migraine and the role of blood vessel constricting (or dilating) amines.

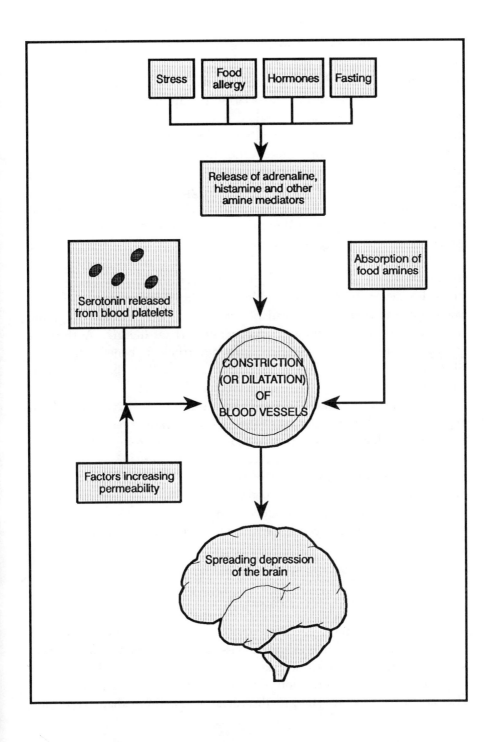

Hormonal changes may predispose to cyclical attacks of migraine in women during the child-bearing years and so can prolonged fasting and a low blood sugar; dietary factors can also be important.

Because of the occasional association of migraine with the classical features of allergy, including a raised serum IgE level, it has often been suggested that migraine is an allergic disorder. As allergic reactions involve a release of histamine, and histamine is known to be a vasodilator capable of precipitating headaches, there is nothing surprising in the concept of allergy as a triggering factor for migraine. In keeping with this, plasma histamine levels have been shown to rise in food-induced migraine (*Mansfield et al., 1985*). An association with other features of allergy is, however, the exception rather than the rule in migraine sufferers and skin tests with foods are usually (but not always) negative. Attention has therefore been focused on biochemical and other factors which may be able to trigger migraine attacks in other ways. On the basis of the available evidence, food-provoked migraine appears to be more commonly biochemical than allergic. A third of patients with severe migraine can nevertheless benefit from an elimination diet. It has been claimed that a few (less than 10%) will become symptom-free (*Vaughan & Mansfield, 1991*).

Other food-provoked neurological symptoms have also been reported. Egger and colleagues (*1983; 1985*) claim that epilepsy can occur in childhood as a reaction to food and that a prolonged remission can be obtained with a restricted diet. Whether this represents a specific effect, or is akin to the traditional treatment of childhood epilepsy using a ketotic diet, remains to be seen. The claim that foods can also cause behavioural disorders in childhood have been discussed in Chapter 3. The special conditions in which this can occur still remain to be established.

The Joints

Inflammatory changes in the joints are a common feature of hypersensitivity reactions, as in the classical example of serum sickness, in which arthritis and kidney damage occur as a part of the immune reaction following the injection of foreign protein. Joint symptoms may also accompany acute allergic disorders of the immediate type; for example, joint pains have been reported in patients with urticaria and angioedema. The knees, wrists and finger joints are the most frequently involved, and there have been a few reports of joint swelling and limitation of movement (*Denman, 1987*). Occasionally, the only manifestation of an apparent hypersensitivity to a food may be pain and swelling of the joints unaccompanied by any other symptoms. It is, however, uncommon to obtain a remission of symptoms by the exclusion of food allergens such as milk, cheese or egg, followed by recurrence during double-blind provocation tests (*Parke & Hughes, 1981*). Panush (*1990*) reported that 30% of their patients with rheumatoid arthritis thought they were worse after specific foods, but only 3 out of 15 who were studied had both a diet-induced remission and a food-induced recurrence during double-blind challenge tests.

The timing of a relapse of joint symptoms – usually 4–24 hours after challenge – does not conform to the usual pattern of IgE-mediated reactions. There have, nevertheless, been occasional cases in which specific foods have appeared to produce an exacerbation of rheumatoid arthritis. Because of this, a number of trials have been carried out in which rheumatoid arthritis has been treated by restrictive diets. In practice, exclusion diets have been found to be of little value (*Denman et al., 1983*). Panush believes that fewer than 5% have any form of food sensitivity.

Whatever the nature of the acute episodes of joint pain provoked by food, they appear to have little relevance to the primary cause of rheumatoid disease. The prevalence of allergic disorders in patients with rheumatoid arthritis and in patients with juvenile chronic arthritis is much the same as in normal control subjects (*Peskett et al., 1981*). In adults with rheumatoid disease, there is no serological evidence of an increase in IgE antibodies to pollens, and the prevalence of IgE antibodies to milk and egg is similar to that of the population in general (*O'Driscoll et al., 1985*). Conversely, the prevalence of rheumatoid arthritis in 266 allergic outpatients was the same as that in the general population.

Attempts to link joint disease with evidence of the immediate type of allergy have thus failed. This is not to deny the potential relationship between food and joint pains, for example, in gout, wherein the onset of painfully swollen joints after rich food and wine can be so dramatic as to be the classical subject of cartoons. However specific this association may appear to be, its relationship is not to immunological change but to uric acid metabolism. When non-gouty subjects complain of joint pains after drinking red wine, it cannot be assumed that the cause is immunological. As food intolerance can have many causes, it may therefore be the metabolic, rather than the immunological, changes that should be studied in patients who develop joint symptoms after specific foods.

The Kidney

In contrast to the lack of evidence for IgE dysfunction as a cause of joint disease, there is clear evidence that, in very occasional cases, allergy can lead to kidney disease. Such cases appear to be rare, but Williams (1987) has documented 17 cases in which the nephrotic syndrome – a kidney disease associated with the leaking of protein into the urine – has been associated with eczema, asthma, or a form of hay fever. There was reasonably good evidence in each case that the association was causal rather than accidental. In six further cases of the nephrotic syndrome (of whom five had other evidence of allergic disease), there was a partial or complete remission on an elemental diet, followed by a relapse on exposure to cow's milk, and a further remission on withdrawal of the milk. There was also a positive skin test to milk. Two other patients were thought to develop protein in the urine in relation to the ingestion of foods (pork and fish in one case, chicken eggs in the other). Although a remission occurred in each case, corticosteroids had been given at the same time as dietary measures were introduced, making it impossible to establish the cause of the remission. Because IgE was not detected in the renal tissue of any of these patients, Williams suggests that the most likely cause of the reaction must involve an indirect effect on the kidney. There may, for example, be a release of substances such as histamine and leukotrienes at other sites in the body which, on reaching the kidney, may produce a change in the permeability of the glomerulus.

The Blood

No discussion of reactions to food would be complete without mention of a very rare complication, provoked by cow's milk, resulting in blood platelet deficiency (thrombocytopenia) in both infants and adults (*Whitfield & Barr, 1976; Caffrey et al., 1981*). As infants with a congenital abnormality associated with bone-marrow deficiency can develop a fall in blood platelet count on drinking cow's milk, it is doubtful if this is an allergic reaction rather than a biochemical one, perhaps associated with platelet 'stickiness'. There is, as yet, no evidence from which to draw firm conclusions concerning this curious condition.

OCCUPATIONAL REACTIONS TO FOOD

An increasing number of chemicals, drugs, wood dusts and other agents used in the manufacturing industries have been shown to cause occupational asthma. Among these are around 50 agents used in food manufacturing (Table 6.7). In many, but not all, cases, there is a family history of allergy, but other factors, such as cigarette-smoking and poor hygiene, may also play a part.

Perhaps the best studied example is 'baker's asthma'. In West Berlin (*Herxheimer, 1967*), serial tests showed an increase from 8% to 30% in positive skin tests to flour in apprentice bakers at the end of a

Table 6.7   Foods capable of causing occupational asthma or rhinitis

● **Fish**	● **Occupation**
Prawn, crab, oysters	Fish-processing
Fishmeal	Factory workers
Mother of pearl	Button manufacturing workers
● **Farm products**	
Cows, pigs, poultry	Farmers
Pheasants, quails	Breeders
Eggs	Egg processors, bakers
● **Plants and fungi**	
Grains, flour	Bakers, millers, food processors
Rice	Rice millers
Soybeans	Agricultural workers
Garlic, spices, tea plant enzymes	Factory workers
Hops	Brewers
Mushrooms	Soup makers

(Modified from *O'Neil & Lehrer, 1991*)

5-year study period. In the former West Germany (*Thiel & Ulmer, 1980*), approximately one-quarter of the 300 bakers per year who claimed occupational disease were awarded compensation.

The diagnosis of occupational asthma is best confirmed by challenge tests and peak flow recordings taken throughout a working week and at the weekends, when an improvement is normally seen. As asthma tends to become worse when exposure continues and may continue long after exposure has stopped, the only practical advice is to change to another type of work.

Apart from asthma, exposure to foods at work can result in a widespread inflammatory process within the lung (hypersensitivity pneumonitis). This is not an immediate allergic reaction, but often presents with fever, chills, cough and malaise, beginning a few hours after exposure and continuing for 18–24 hours or more. Although this may represent a reaction to the food itself, it is more usually the result of contamination by mites, bacteria, fungi or other extraneous substances (Table 6.8). The interstices of the lung become infiltrated with inflammatory cells – mostly lymphocytes – and, although the blood contains antibodies which can react with the food, they are of the IgG class – and therefore capable of forming immune complexes – rather than IgE. This IgG response may well be a reaction provoked by the contaminants as well as the food, but it may not be the immediate cause of the lung reaction. On the basis of the evidence, it appears probable that the hypersensitivity pneumonitis which occurs is the result of the delayed type 4 reaction (see Chapter 5; Table 5.1), possibly with some damage due to immune complexes (type 3). As the condition tends to progress, a change of occupation is the only satisfactory approach.

Table 6.8 Hypersensitivity pneumonitis in the food industries

Examples of agents	Examples of diseases
Moulds in hay, barley, malt, sugar cane, compost, cheese, grapes	Farmer's lung, malt-worker's lung, cheese-worker's lung
Weevils, mites in grains, cheese	Miller's lung, cheese-worker's lung
Duck, chicken, turkey or goose proteins (or feathers)	Feather-plucker's disease, turkey-handler's disease

(Modified from *O'Neil & Lehrer, 1991*)

Contact dermatitis is also a hazard in some industries; in some cases, urticarial weals or a more widespread eczema can develop (Table 6.9). Bakers who have skin disease may not, however, be reacting to flour alone. Irritant reactions to wet sticky dough, emulsifiers, bleaching agents and various chemicals and yeast can all occur. True allergic reactions can also develop against a number of flavouring materials and chemicals, such as sorbic acid. Skin patch tests, using a battery of substances strapped to the skin, can produce diagnostic evidence which may help to pinpoint one or two substances to be avoided.

Management of Adverse Reactions

Occupational reactions to foods present a different type of problem from the adverse reactions encountered in the population at large. Whatever the type of reaction encountered in a non-industrial setting, the first objective is to identify the cause of the reaction beyond any doubt, and the aim of treatment is then to eliminate the appropriate foods from the diet. There may be difficulties if the food is widely used in cooking (milk, egg, wheat, flour), or if a common preservative or colouring agent is involved. Furthermore, a restricted diet, especially in children deprived of cow's milk, may lead to calcium and vitamin deficiencies unless appropriate supplements are given. A dietician's advice is therefore required.

Table 6.9   Dermatitis in the food industry

Processes and foods involved	Main skin problem
Handlers of cow's milk	Contact dermatitis
Cooks using mustard, garlic, onions	Eczema
Other food workers	Contact dermatitis
Bakers	Contact dermatitis/eczema
Butchers, poulterers	Urticaria, eczema
Fishermen, fish handlers, factory workers	Contact urticaria, contact dermatitis

(Modified from *O'Neil & Lehrer, 1991*)

In infants with cow's milk-protein intolerance, the use of protein hydrolysates can be helpful, although their expense and unpleasant taste may make such a regime difficult to sustain. The use of soya milk, appropriately fortified with vitamins, or goat's or sheep's milk can occasionally be of value, although each in itself can provoke occasional allergic reactions. It should be remembered that intolerance to some soya-milk preparations is related to the added sugar rather than to the soya.

In the most severe cases, elemental diets have been used for short periods, but it is doubtful whether restrictions of this kind are indicated except for diagnosis, when such a diet may be necessary to satisfy both the patient and the relatives that a previously made diagnosis of food intolerance cannot be substantiated.

The treatment of associated allergies is also important. A patient who has both a food allergy and an associated asthma or eczema may react less severely to foods after the associated allergies have been successfully treated. The management of asthma is the subject of monographs, and involves the problems of lifestyle, antigen avoidance and hyposensitization, and pharmacological approaches involving cromolyns, bronchodilators, and topical or systemic corticosteroids.

Treatment of the child with eczema has already been discussed (see page 95), including the need to replace soap with an aqueous cream or an oatmeal-based preparation. Similar methods are equally appropriate for adults. Bath additives containing oat protein and the use of emulsifying ointment after bathing can prevent the skin from drying. The use of primrose oil and other vegetable compounds have shown promise, but these are still under evaluation (*Galloway et al., 1991*). Where necessary, topical corticosteroids can be used, preferably in their least potent form and for the shortest period possible. If secondary infection requires the use of antibiotics, these should be given orally for short periods to reduce the risk of skin sensitization or the development of resistant organisms. Cotton stockings or mittens can help to reduce scratching during sleep.

Pharmacological treatment of the food allergy itself is virtually confined to the treatment of symptoms or to the emergency treatment of anaphylaxis. The prophylactic use of oral disodium cromoglycate has been widely advocated, but it is not equally effective in all cases. Aspirin and other non-steroidal anti-inflammatory drugs (NSAIDs) have also been used in the symptomatic treatment of food-induced bouts of sneezing, and in the treatment of diarrhoea and other gastrointestinal reactions. The effect is presumed to be non-specific, as cyclooxygenase inhibitors can sometimes relieve diarrhoea due to a variety of other causes (*Buisseret et al., 1978*).

Attempts at desensitization have been popular among practitioners of alternative medicine, but such claims have been discredited by a failure to produce sound evidence of efficacy. Hopes have been raised by Shenassa and colleagues (*1985*), who claimed to have studied four patients who lost their anaphylactic reactivity to peanut after a prolonged course of oral desensitization. Some support for these claims has been provided by Bullock (*1992*), but the method carries the danger of severe anaphylactic reactions during treatment and does not appear to provide a reliable solution to the problem.

Dietary restriction thus remains the mainstay of treatment, provided that the culprit food or foods have been positively identified. The simplest approach is to eliminate a particular suspect food — for example, strawberries or shellfish — but, if a more stringent elimination diet is necessary, a dietitian's help should be obtained to ensure the adequacy of calories, protein, calcium and vitamins.

Where an allergic food reaction is suspected, a simple exclusion diet can be used (Table 6.10). With the possible exception of gluten-free bread, which can be omitted if necessary, the ingredients are easily

Table 6.10 Simple exclusion diet

Permitted	Major exclusions
Lamb, mutton	Other meat, poultry, fish
Gluten-free bread Rice, rice products[a]	Other bread, cakes, biscuits, pasta, cereals
Vegetarian margarine	Milk, butter, dairy products, eggs
Fresh fruit, vegetables	Nuts, strawberries, preserves, commercially frozen foods
Tea, coffee, fresh fruit juices	Wines, spirits
Sugar, barley sugar	Confectionery
Olive oil	

[a] Except in rice-eating countries, where the possibility of reactions to rice should be borne in mind.

available. It also has the practical advantage that it can be followed without difficulty on an outpatient basis for a period of 1–2 weeks or longer, if necessary. If the symptoms disappear, the suggestion that dietary factors have been involved is strengthened. There is still a need, however, to demonstrate that a patient who remains well on such a diet will have a recurrence of symptoms when a new food is added. A succession of new foods are therefore introduced, each one being taken in reasonably large quantities for a period of a few days. If the symptoms return, the most recently added food is suspected to be the cause and more formal challenge tests can then be initiated. The results help to establish whether particular foods should be avoided over a longer period.

Should the initial diet fail to relieve symptoms, it may be reasonable to reassure the patient of the need for long-term dietary measures, unless there is circumstantial evidence of food intolerance sufficiently strong to justify further efforts. In such a case, there is the alternative of removing one or two suspect foods for a further 1–2 weeks or, alternatively, changing a few ingredients in the empirical diet along the lines shown in Table 6.11. As noted earlier, it is exceptional for the use of an elemental diet to be justified.

The above recommendations apply especially to patients whose symptoms occur shortly after food is taken and especially if there are symptoms which suggest an allergic reaction. If the symptoms are delayed and confined to the digestive tract, an allergic cause is unlikely,

Table 6.11 Exclusion diet alternative ingredients

Permitted	Substituting for
Beef or chicken	Lamb, mutton
Tapioca; rye crispbread, maize, corn flakes (after 3-day interval)	Gluten-free bread, rice
Carrots, lettuce, potatoes (as before)	Exclude peas, beans, soya
Most soft fruits (as before)	Exclude citrus fruits, apples
Water	Tea, coffee, fruit juice
Corn oil, sunflower or cottonseed oil	Olive oil
Corn syrup	Sugar

and the initial dietary regime can be modified. Although milk, eggs, cereal foods (including gluten-free bread), coffee and tea should still be excluded, there is little likelihood that fish or processed meat are responsible, and these foods can be allowed. It may be advisable, however, to exclude citrus fruits and fresh vegetables during the first week. In a study of 200 patients with the irritable bowel syndrome the majority (156) of whom had symptoms for over 2 years, 91 improved on a restricted diet and, of these, 73 were able to identify one or more foods which provoked a recurrence of their symptoms (*Nanda et al., 1989*). Of these patients, 72 remained well on a modified diet for an average follow-up period of 14.7 months.

When a diet is finally established on which the patient can remain symptom-free, it should be borne in mind that partial or complete tolerance to a food may develop over time, especially in young children. Except in the most severe cases, the reintroduction of a food may therefore be considered on a trial basis after an interval of a few months. In severe cases, the deliberate or accidental reintroduction of a food may carry risks, however; should anaphylactic reactions occur, patients may need to be given a subcutaneous or intramuscular injection of adrenaline (epinephrine) supported by oral or injected corticosteroids and antihistamines.

In the less severe cases of food intolerance, occasional dietary indiscretions cause only minor problems which tend to diminish. Some persist, and various types of nuts, sesame seeds, mustard, spices, and fruits have been shown to provoke recurrent anaphylactic reactions that show few signs of abatement over many years. Other foods causing recurrent anaphylaxis after long intervals include milk, to which, however, tolerance is more likely to develop.

There are no fixed rules as to the length of time that a strict exclusion diet be pursued in a highly allergic subject. Childhood allergy to egg – to take one example – usually remits. The reintroduction of small amounts of food containing cooked egg is therefore justified within a few months in a child with egg-provoked eczema. It should be noted, however, that patients who exhibit the less immediate type of reaction may appear to tolerate a single challenge but will suffer cumulative effects if egg, milk, or other relevant foods are given in large quantities or on frequent occasions. Eczema patients who are allergic to egg sometimes insist that they can tolerate foods containing egg with impunity, provided that they take them no more frequently than once or twice weekly. Others maintain that egg or milk that has been denatured by prolonged cooking causes no problems, but will provoke symptoms when given in other forms.

CONCLUSION

The diagnosis of food intolerance can only be proved by a clinical challenge test in which the food is given in a form which cannot be identified by the patient. For clinical purposes, a history of repeated anaphylactic reactions may make this unnecessary or even dangerous. A positive skin-prick test or IgE blood test can also provide supporting evidence for the diagnosis of food allergy.

The majority of problems arise in children, especially in infants with cow's milk-protein intolerance, and there is evidence that the intestinal mucosa can be damaged in these cases. Potentiating factors may operate in malnourished children or in rotavirus infections. Eczema and asthma are among the other manifestations in childhood.

Even in childhood, food intolerance is not always associated with allergy. In adults, non-immunological mechanisms are more in evidence, especially in cases where larger quantities of food lead to intestinal reactions after a delay of several hours. Other syndromes can arise, including food-provoked migraine and, in occasional cases, joint pains and kidney disease.

CHAPTER

——7——

Food Additives

The contribution of the media to health education has been, at times, very positive but, at other times, uncritical and harmful. Alongside highly responsible and widely admired reporters, there are those who give wide publicity to maverick claims or untested remedies, and who advocate sensational new cancer cures in Switzerland, treatment for 'total allergy' in the United States, the cure of obesity through the use of cytotoxic food allergy tests or the solution to childhood behaviour disorders through the banning of food additives of almost every kind. As far as food nutrition and dietary fads are concerned, the fashionable nostrums that have boosted vitamin crazes in the United States, and warned us about low blood sugar or the poisonous effects of food additives, have been fuelled by uncritical publicity on a major scale. Without an effective body to maintain ethical standards or to discipline malpractice, the power of television, radio and the press is virtually unrestrained. However, as always, the issues raised by the media are worthy of debate. The position of food additives therefore deserves critical examination.

WHAT ARE THEY?

A food additive is defined as a substance that is not commonly regarded or used as food, but which is added to, or used in or on, food at any stage for purposes of maintaining quality, texture, consistency, taste, odour, alkalinity or acidity, or to serve any other technological function in relation to food; this includes processing aids insofar as they are added to, or used in or on, food (*Food Labelling Regulations, 1984*). In other words, they include a wide range of substances that make a food look, taste or smell better, or improve its texture or keeping qualities (Table 7.1). Additives should therefore not be regarded as a single group of substances, whether for general approval or condemnation. Some could be omitted without difficulty, but food distribution would be seriously threatened without preservatives to prevent bacterial or fungal contamination, or without agents that prevent food from deteriorating and becoming rancid. Sulphites are not only preservatives, but also prevent enzymatic browning in vegetables and fruit. Sodium nitrite inhibits the growth of *Clostridium botulinum* spores in cured meats. The growth of moulds is prevented by calcium propionate in bread and sorbic acid in drinks.

The merits and disadvantages of each of these substances should be considered separately. A regulating authority, therefore, must evaluate approximately 350 antioxidants, colours, preservatives and other miscellaneous additives in addition to perhaps 3000–4000 flavouring substances, some of which are still under examination. Added to these are contaminants acquired at an earlier stage of food production, for example, pesticide and veterinary drug residues (*Munro, 1986*), which need to be kept under surveillance.

Table 7.1 Types of food additives

Main function	Additive category
Keeping properties	Preservatives
	Antioxidants
	Sequestrants
Keeping properties and flavour	Acidity regulators
Improved flavour	Flavours and flavour potentiators
	Sweeteners
Improved appearance	Colours
	Glazes
Modified consistency and texture	Emulsifiers
	Stabilizers
	Thickeners

(Modified from *Smith et al., 1991*)

Food additives ensure the safety of foods but are also concerned with convenience, attractiveness, and achieving a consistent appearance and quality. Both the EEC Scientific Committee for Food and the United Nations Joint Expert Committee on Food Additives are concerned with assessing whether new ingredients are needed and whether they are safe. No substances can be generally introduced until this approval is given.

In the United States, many widely used substances have slowly acquired 'grandfather status' (generally recognized as safe). Some of these substances occur naturally. Benzoic acid, which is added to carbonated drinks to prevent microbial spoilage, can be found in cranberries and a variety of other foods. Sorbic acid can be used for the same purpose. Lecithin, which adds stability to salad dressings and cake mixes, is found in egg yolks and soybeans; and proteolytic enzymes used, for example, as meat tenderizers, are obtainable from papaya (papain), pineapple (bromelain), bovine pancreas (trypsin) and abomasum (pepsin) (*Levine et al., 1985*). In the United Kingdom, there is a requirement to carry out extensive tests upon new additives in the regulated categories to establish their technological need and safety. Existing additives are also reviewed in the light of any new information on toxicology, changing levels of exposure, or risk assessments derived from both chemical and clinical information.

Complaints about food additives are chiefly concerned with their safety. Questions are also raised as to the need for 'cosmetic' additives, such as colourings, and concerning the appropriateness of using flavouring or bulking agents that disguise or dilute food products. Those who complain, whether justifiably or not, can point to a marked increase in the use of additives between 1955 and 1985. It is estimated that each person consumes 6–11 lb of additives each year (*Association of County Councils Publications, 1987*). Concerns about food additive intolerance were expressed in the European Community Reports of the Scientific Committee for Food (*1982*). In the United Kingdom, this was followed by the publication of the Labelling in Food Regulations (*1984*), which set out requirements for the specific declaration of antioxidants, colouring matter, emulsifiers, stabilizers, mineral hydrocarbons, preservatives, solvents, sweeteners, and a host of miscellaneous antifoaming and anticaking agents, flavour modifiers (but not flavouring agents), flour bleachers and improvers, bulking agents and liquid freezants. By July 1986, all additives had to be listed by name or code number on the wrappers of purchased food (Table 7.2) and, as a result, many members of the public became aware of their presence for the first time.

It is of interest that the introduction of these public-spirited measures served to arouse anxieties rather than allay them. There followed a lively debate on the value of food additives and, at least in Great Britain, particular disdain was apparently attached to code numbers with the prefix 'E' (denoting approval by the European Community). When a food company asked housewives if they would buy a product (in fact, spinach) which contained water, vegetable protein and oil, sugars, oxalic acid, the colours E140 and E160, and preservatives E250 and E251, many said they would not. The conclusion drawn was that E numbers were a disincentive to purchase and, noting this, some manufacturers substituted seminatural sub-stances, such as caramelized sugar. There is no evidence that such policies result in a safer product. Concern over E numbers nevertheless persists, and food labels tend to refer to citric acid and ascorbic acid by name rather than as E330 and E300.

Toxicological data on food additives are widely available to regulating authorities and will not be further considered here. Public concern over additive-induced reactions in susceptible subjects remains, however, substantial. Reports of adverse reactions to additives in medicine (*Lockey, 1959*) have also been a cause for comment, and have been the subject of consultations between the Department of Health

Table 7.2 Additive categories given European Community approval

Category	Example	E number
Colours	Tumeric, tartrazine, titanium dioxide	E100–E180
Preservatives	Benzoates, sulphites	E200–E290
Antioxidants	Vitamin C, butylated hydroxyanisole and hydroxytoluene	E300–E321
Emulsifiers Stabilizers Sweeteners	Lecithin, carrageenan, sorbitol	E322–E495

and pharmaceutical companies in the United Kingdom (*Association of County Councils Publications, 1987*). Judging from the continuing widespread use of benzoates, sorbates, sunset yellow and erythrosine in medicinal preparations (*Frei, 1989*), however, there has, as yet, been little change in manufacturers' practices. The use of tartrazine appears to be the exception and has steadily declined.

HOW DID THE USE OF ADDITIVES DEVELOP?

Concerns about food preservation are not new, but have arisen whenever food supplies have increased above subsistence level. As the natural shelf-life of most foods is very short, traditional attempts to salt or pickle foods or to process them in other ways, for example, by burying them underground (as in *grav lux*), have been of great importance and were the forerunners of food technology.

In more modern times, further advances have developed not only from the need to prevent famine or to stretch food supplies during the winter months, but also in response to an unexpected stimulus arising from the wish to feed large armies. The heat preservation of food in glass bottles was developed by Nicholas Appet of France in 1811 as a means of helping Napoleon to feed his troops (*Levine et al., 1985*). This method preceded any knowledge of bacterial, fungal, physical, chemical or enzyme-induced decay. Within 50 years, the glass bottles had been replaced by tin canisters, and mechanical refrigeration was also being introduced, making it possible to ship meat over long distances. By the time of World War I, the monotony of 'bully beef' in tins had become the butt of music-hall jokes.

In due course, new standards for food preservation were set. Various types of heat treatment, methods of dehydration, and the removal of tissue gases provided additional techniques, and the use of food additives were among the many methods developed to improve keeping qualities and prevent deterioration.

An indirect means of preserving food is by altering its water content, as water is needed for the microbial, chemical and enzymatic reactions that can damage food. These damaging reactions are stopped by processes which make water unavailable, such as freezing or drying, and other processes are useful even when water is only partially removed, for example, when foods are smoked, baked, or fried in deep fat. Humectants – chemicals that bind water – have a similar effect by making the water less available, and include sucrose, glucose, fructose, sodium chloride and propylene glycol. As in the traditional methods of pickling, the empirical use of humectants began before the term was invented – indeed, before the science of food technology was even conceived. Jams and jellies have made use of humectants long before they were classified as food additives or included in this controversial category.

A further method for inhibiting the growth of microbes depends on processes involving fermentation, and uses yeast or other organisms selected for their ability to alter the acidity or alcohol content of food. Fermentation has its chief importance in making wine, beer, cheese, bread and vinegar, and in the preservation of olives and pickles. The processes employed also make use of a number of miscellaneous additives; for example, in traditional wine-making processes, sodium metabisulphite is used to kill the yeast and stop fermentation at the appropriate time. The highest concentrations are often found in the finest clarets. Sodium stearyl-lactylate, a naturally occurring compound, has long been added to bread to delay the stale hardening of starch which otherwise occurs. Calcium propionate is also added to bread to prevent the growth of spoilage moulds.

Despite these benign examples of food processing, in the past suspicions concerning the substances added to food have undoubtedly been justified. In the nineteenth century, the unregulated use of added substances allowed widespread adulteration of food. In the United States, chalk was added to watered milk, and copper salts were added to canned vegetables to make them look green (*Levine et al., 1985*). Public pressure led to the United Kingdom Pure Food and Drug Act of 1906, and successive extensions have helped to regulate the use of substances added to food or medicine. When the United States Army introduced the irradiation of food in 1957, this form of 'cold sterilization' was classed as a food additive, with the intention that each irradiated food should then be tested for toxicity.

REGULATIONS ON FOOD ADDITIVES

The present position is that no new additive may be introduced in the United Kingdom, Europe or the United States without first demonstrating efficacy and a reasonable case for using it, after which its biological safety must be demonstrated by means which are clearly laid down, and are both expensive and time-consuming. Long-term feeding studies are required in animals for 2–3 years, with specific tests for possible effects on reproduction and on the potential damage to offspring. Food-additive testing inevitably takes several years before a new product can be introduced and is likely to cost several millions of pounds.

EXAMPLES OF ADDITIVES IN CURRENT USE

The colouring materials used in food have changed considerably since 1857, when it was not unknown for sweets to be coloured by red lead, lead chromate, mercuric sulphide or copper arsenate (*David, 1988*). While most of the additives in current use have other purposes, colours still account for many of the most widely used agents.

By far the best known of the additives in current use is the colouring agent tartrazine (E102), a yellow coal-tar dye which is sometimes mixed with other coal-tar dyes, such as sunset yellow (E110), amaranth red (E123) or brilliant blue FCF (133) to produce shades of cream, orange or green. It is incorporated into thousands of food products, especially drinks, sweets, pastries and sauces. Many other coal-tar dyes are in use – for example, erythrosine (E127), around 60 tons of which are used annually in the United States.

Colours have also been used in an attempt to mimic a natural appearance. Until recently, it was customary to stain kippers brown, but this practice is waning. The colour of fresh, farmed salmon is due to added cantaxanthin, which is used to replace the astaxanthin obtained by salmon in the wild from crustacea in their natural diet. The colour of mozzarella cheese (with the exception of buffalo mozzarella) is derived from titanium oxide, which may be added in quantities up to 400 mg/kg.

A number of other colouring materials have attracted attention because they are naturally occurring, including cochineal, a well-known household colouring material derived from the *Coccus cacti* beetle of South America. Other 'natural' substances include chlorophyll, annatto (from the tree), yellow, orange and red carotenes, paprika products, and caramel (burnt sugar). It is still unclear whether they have advantages because they are of natural origin, but their method of production is not simple; for example, there are now at least 100 different commercially available caramels, which the International Caramel Manufacturers' organization categorize as caustic caramel, caustic sulphite caramel, ammonia caramel and ammonium sulphite caramel. Manufacturers now use the caramels more widely than any other colouring agent, especially in beers, wine, whiskies, bread and biscuits. With the increased popularity of brown bread, flour which has been whitened may even have caramel added to make it brown again.

The preservatives provide another large and important category of additives by helping to prevent food decay and the spread of food-borne infection. This group includes substances which have been used traditionally for a very long time, for example, the sorbic acid derivatives (E200–203) used widely in cakes and baked foods, benzoic acid and benzoates (E210–E219) used mainly in processed fruits, jams, jellies and soft drinks, and sulphur dioxide and sulphiting agents (E221–E227), now the most widely used antimicrobial preservatives. These substances prevent the growth of undesirable microorganisms in the fermentation industry and, perhaps not surprisingly, are consumed in the largest quantities by heavy wine drinkers (Table 7.3).

The popularity of the sulphiting agents has depended, for 100 years or more, on their additional ability to prevent oxidation in oils and fats and the brown discoloration of foods caused by enzymes, and their overall success in preserving the appearance and flavour of foods. Of the other preservatives in use, the nitrates (E249–E252) help to give preserved meats their pink colour. Acetic acid (E260) is the traditional main ingredient of vinegar and of many pickling processes, and other acetates may be used in frozen vegetables and soups. Propionic acid and

Table 7.3 Daily estimated intake of sulphites

	Mean daily intake (mg)	Plus 350 ml of wine
Belgium	8–10	144
Germany	9–10	144
Switzerland	4.2	–

(Modified from *Frei, 1989*)

propionates (E280–E283) are antimould agents used in bread, baked goods and some cheeses.

Antioxidants extend the shelf life of foods and prevent fats from going rancid. Vitamin C (ascorbic acid, E300) is widely used for this purpose, and may be combined with other more effective, synthetic substances, such as butylated hydroxyanisole (E320), butylated hydroxytoluene (E321), and octyl and dodecyl gallate (E311, E312). The other categories of food additives include the emulsifiers and stabilizers (including stearyl-lactylate used in bread), and thickeners, such as agar, various gums, and carrageenan. Some sweeteners also have bulking properties (sorbitol and glycerol), and there are a variety of acids, bases, intense sweeteners, solvents, and glazing, bleaching and anticaking agents.

Flavour-enhancing agents deserve special mention because of the importance of glutamic acid and monosodium glutamate (620, 621), which are present in around 10,000 processed foods in the United States, and consumed in quantities which can amount to an individual intake of several pounds of monosodium glutamate a year. As a naturally occurring amino acid, its safety in use has been assumed, but questions have been raised concerning its capacity to produce clinical symptoms at the concentrations in which it is often taken (see below).

Table 7.4 provides a few examples of the categories of food in which particular types of additive may be found. As there are several additives in a simple loaf of bread, this table represents a considerable simplification.

DO ADDITIVES CAUSE UNPLEASANT REACTIONS?

Suspicions concerning the toxic effects of food additives are not new. 'Tell your grocer and butcher,' wrote Dr H. W. Wiley in 1913, 'you will take no more fruits, molasses, sirups or meats that contain sulphurous acid or sulphites' (Sloan & Powers, 1986). Indeed, it is now generally accepted that sulphites can provoke asthmatic attacks (Bush et al., 1986).

Sulphites

In the case of sulphiting agents, the results of investigations are no longer controversial. These substances, when added as preservatives to both foods and medicines, have been reported to cause flushing, throat-swelling, itching of the mouth and skin, and asthma in a substantial

Table 7.4 Examples of additive-containing foods

Additive category	Examples of use
Colours	Tinned and packeted convenience foods
	Jams, sauces, drinks, soups, confectionery
Preservatives	
Sorbic acid	Cakes and baked foods
Benzoates	Fruit products, soft drinks, pickles, sauces, salad dressings
Sulphites	Dried fruits, various drinks, sausages, processed potatoes, shrimps
Nitrates	Cooked and cured meats and sausages
Propionic acid	Baked food and dairy products
Antioxidants	
Ascorbic acid (vitamin C)	Fruit juices, bread and baked produce
Butylated hydroxyanisole + hydroxytoluene (BHA, BHT)	Crisps, biscuits, pastry, bottled sauces, fried foods
Emulsifiers and stabilizers	
Lecithins	Chocolate products, powdered milk, margarine
Alginates and agar	Ice cream, jellies, instant desserts and puddings
Celluloses	High-fibre bread and low-calorie produce
Fatty-acid products	Powdered milk, soups, bread and baked products

number of cases (*Koepke et al., 1984*; *Gibson & Clancy 1980*; *Stephenson & Simon, 1981*). Salad components, such as lettuce, retain nearly all of the added sulphite in its free form and have been shown to be potent triggers of asthma (*Taylor et al., 1986*). These and other sulphite-containing foods can provoke anything from mild wheezing to life-threatening asthma episodes in about 5% of the asthmatic population (*Simon, 1989*). Indeed, inhaled sulphur dioxide at a concentration of one part per million can be enough to cause wheezing (*Boughey, 1982*). In the United States, the Food and Drug Administration has now banned the use of sulphites on fruits and vegetables served as fresh but they are still encountered in dried fruit, beer and wine, sausages, processed potato, pickles and shrimps. Their use in nebulized drugs can also cause problems.

It has been suggested that sulphites cause problems only in solution (*Towns & Mellis, 1984*), especially if that solution is acidic. Asthma can also be provoked, however, by the injection of sulphite-containing drug solutions. Allen and Delohery (1985) carried out an experiment in which sodium metabisulphite in solution was swilled around the mouth with impunity, so long as the subject stopped breathing. Without breath-holding, an identical test in a susceptible subject appeared to produce an asthmatic attack. By implication, it was the inhaling of sulphur dioxide fumes that triggered asthma in such individuals, a conclusion endorsed by Bush and co-workers (1986). This may help to explain the variable response to a metabisulphite challenge, even in cases where there is a convincing history of sulphite-related asthmatic attacks. It is also possible that different substances potentiate the effects of one another. When four asthmatics were observed by Gershwin and colleagues to have asthmatic reactions after drinking wine, a disguised drink containing alcohol provoked asthma in one subject, and another reacted to a similarly flavoured drink containing sodium metabisulphite. Each substance was thus shown to be able to provoke asthma in individual cases, but the combined effects of both was not studied.

Concern has also been voiced over a number of other substances. In addition to sulphites, Simon (1989) lists sodium benzoate, coal-tar dyes, nitrates, monosodium glutamate, butylated hydroxyanisole and hydroxytoluene, and the sweetener aspartame as potential causes of reactions.

Benzoates and Parabens

Numerous studies have shown that benzoates can provoke symptoms in patients with chronic urticaria. The prevalence of intolerance to benzoates in this group of subjects has been reported to be as high as 10–20%. It is now clear that a number of non-specific stimuli can provoke attacks in susceptible individuals but, when challenge tests are given blind and the results compared with the effects of a placebo substance, far fewer positive results are obtained (Jacobsen, 1991). Benzoates can also provoke asthma, but this is uncommon.

The related paraben family of food additives has occasionally been shown to provoke similar symptoms. They are, however, frequently used as preservatives in pharmaceutical skin preparations and cosmetics. In this role, they can sometimes cause contact dermatitis. Benzoates and sorbic acid have also been known to cause local reactions on contact with the skin, especially in children who smear food around their faces (*Clemmensen & Hjorth, 1982*).

Coal-Tar Dyes

Tartrazine is the best known of a group of coal-tar derivatives, which include the azo dyes ponceau, sunset yellow and amaranth, and the non-azo dyes brilliant blue and erythrosine.

The role of tartrazine in provoking urticaria has been confirmed in double-blind studies (*Settipane et al., 1976*) but, of all patients with chronic urticaria, it is unlikely that more than approximately one in 25 cases is due to this cause (*Simon, 1989*). Most investigators consider this figure much too high. Murdoch and colleagues (*1987*) were able to find only two cases in which urticaria was provoked by tartrazine or other azo dyes. While accepting that tartrazine can produce such effects, Stevenson and colleagues (*1986*) suggest that the relationship between tartrazine and asthma is dubious, and double-blind trials with allegedly tartrazine-sensitive asthmatics have been unconvincing. In Sweden, where the use of tartrazine has been banned, evidence is still needed as to whether this exclusion policy has led to any change in the prevalence of such reactions as urticaria, asthma or childhood behavioural disorders, which have sometimes been claimed to be a consequence of the ingestion of tartrazine.

Monosodium Glutamate

Seaweeds have traditionally been used in Asia to enhance the flavour of food, and monosodium glutamate has been ascertained to be the active ingredient responsible for this effect. As glutamic acid is abundant in many foods and is one of the natural amino acids from which proteins are built, monosodium glutamate has generally been regarded as safe. When large amounts of dissolved glutamate are taken on an empty stomach, however, the evidence strongly suggests that it can cause asthma and other symptoms.

The 'Chinese restaurant syndrome' has been much discussed since its first description by Kwok in 1968 (*Smith et al., 1982*; *Allen, 1991*) and may be much less common that was, at first, believed (see p.139). Chest tightness, nausea, a burning sensation of the face and neck, headaches and sweating have all been described. These symptoms can be reproduced by 3 grams or less of free monosodium glutamate (*Schaumberg et al., 1969*), an amount which may be present in an average helping of wonton soup.

It is still not clear whether this is a specific entity or whether, as suggested by Price and colleagues (*1978*), it arises from a non-specific form of oesophageal irritation which could equally well be produced by spiced tomato juice. Headache and bloating may also occur, but this could be related to meals with a high sodium content. The mechanism by which asthma is provoked (*Allen et al., 1987*) may also be different, especially as both early and late reactions have been described.

Aspartame

In the case of aspartame, public concern was aroused by a number of newspaper articles supported by a report of two cases of urticaria (*Kulczycki, 1986*). A determined further search over a period of 32 months, however, has been unable to identify a single case (*Garriga et al., 1991*). During this period, 61 individuals either self-referred or referred by a physician, were carefully screened as it was suggested that the patient was suffering from aspartame-provoked symptoms. None of these suspicions was confirmed.

Other Additives

Butylated hydroxyanisole and butylated hydroxytoluene are antioxidant food preservatives that can aggravate urticaria in occasional cases (*Goodman et al., 1990*). Sodium nitrite is reported to produce dilatation of blood vessels, thereby causing headache, skin rashes and gastrointestinal symptoms at a dose of 20 mg, which is within the range encountered in food (*Moneret-Vautrin et al., 1980*). Proteolytic enzymes used as meat tenderizers have also come under examination (*Levine et al., 1985*). A number of flavouring substances have been thought to exacerbate a preexisting eczema (Table 7.5), especially the balsams and resins, which may occur naturally in food, as well as other flavouring agents, many of them also naturally occurring, such as cinnamon, vanilla, lovage and certain oils (juniper, spearmint, caraway seed) (*Cronin, 1980; Veien et al., 1985*).

Table 7.5 Food flavourings causing exacerbations of eczema

Balsams, resins (including ginger resinoid)
Cinnamon
Vanilla
Lovage
Oils of juniper, spearmint, caraway

Suspect foods
  Beverages (balsam, lovage)
  Chocolate
  Orange peel
  Vanilla or cinnamon flavours, as in ice cream,
    toothpaste
  Foods with oil of juniper (e.g. sausage)
  Lovage-containing food, confectionery, drugs, tobacco

(Reviewed by *Cronin, 1980*; *Veien et al., 1985*)

Ironically, an obsession with 'natural' foods has sometimes diverted attention from the natural foods which contain toxic substances. Their potential for causing harm should not be exaggerated, but we should be aware of the oxalic acid in rhubarb, the cyanogens in almonds and lima beans, the goitre-provoking potential in brassica, the light-sensitizing psoralens in celery, peas and parsley, and the lectins in red kidney beans.

Regulating Additive Usage

From the point of view of a regulating authority, it is necessary to establish that additives are safe for the population at large and in the concentrations in which they are generally used, while accepting that there could still be individuals who react adversely. In practice, this tends to be achieved by establishing a 'no-effect' level, then allowing a safety factor of at least 10, with much higher safety factors in some cases (*Munro, 1986*). While ensuring a high degree of safety for the population at large, these safety measures cannot ensure that susceptible people will not be at risk on occasions. It should be pointed out, however, that the available evidence suggests that their risk is considerably less than the risk of reacting to common foods which contain no additives at all.

Government policies have therefore encouraged the identification of food ingredients by food-labelling but, provided that general safety standards are met, have not suggested the banning of substances which may occasionally cause reactions in a small minority of people.

CONFIRMING CLINICAL SUSPICIONS

Paradoxically, there has been difficulty in reproducing challenge test results consistently, even in subjects with tartrazine reactions diagnosed by double-blind testing (*Gibson & Clancy, 1980*). After initial challenge tests have given positive results, the patient's reactivity often appears to wane or even disappears. It has also been noted that the administration of the challenge material may need to be combined with other potentiating factors before the reaction becomes manifest, as in the asthma studies of Wilson and colleagues (*1982*) reported in Chapter 6. The role of potentiating factors is not only seen in reactions to food additives, but also in reactions to natural foods and, furthermore, not only in reactions with a biochemical basis, but also in those which are clearly allergic. As noted earlier, patients who have IgE antibodies to foods may fail to react on some occasions, but may have severe or even dangerous reactions on exercising after eating (*Maulitz et al., 1979*; *Kidd et al., 1983*). Negative challenge tests in laboratory conditions may not, therefore, be sufficient to exclude food or food-additive sensitivity.

In the case of food additives, there are also other factors to consider, such as the possibility that absorption of these substances can vary, or that their metabolism can be altered by foods taken at the same time (as happens when monosodium glutamate and carbohydrate are taken together (*Allen, 1991*)). The absorption of small molecules is known to rise sharply during bouts of viral gastroenteritis (*Noone et al., 1986*). The limited absorption of tartrazine, usually at around 4%, could therefore be influenced by changes in intestinal permeability. It may be important to establish whether variations in the absorption of an additive such as tartrazine can modify an individual's liability to develop an adverse response.

While bearing in mind the vagaries of the clinical response rate, attempts have been made to increase the sensitivity of challenge tests by measuring not only IgE antibodies, but also the release of inflammatory mediators during the course of the challenge procedure. One outcome has been the demonstration that the reactions which occur are not uncommonly pseudoallergic, and that even urticaria and asthma may be unaccompanied by evidence of an IgE response or any other immunological mechanism. Although IgE-mediated reactions to food additives can occur – for example, to papain used as a meat tenderizer (*Mansfield & Bowers, 1983*) – they appear to be less frequent than direct toxic effects (for example, asthma caused by inhaled sulphur dioxide) or pharmacological effects (for example, vasodilatation caused by nitrites). Adverse effects may also be caused by enzyme deficiencies; for example, the dye orange-RN (prohibited in Europe) is selectively toxic in individuals who lack the enzyme glucose-6-phosphate dehydrogenase (*Akinyanju & Odusote, 1983*).

A similar clinical outcome can thus be triggered by different mechanisms. In place of the search for unidentified immunological abnormalities, increasing efforts have been directed towards the evidence that mediators, such as histamine, are released in the body (*Heatley et al., 1982*), or that a food can make a child more susceptible to the non-specific triggering of bronchospasm by inhaled amounts of bronchoconstricting substances (*Wilson et al., 1982*).

Estimates of Prevalence

Population surveys at High Wycombe have shown that adverse reactions to common foods occur in 1.4–1.9% of the population (*Young,* unpublished report), and may therefore be more than 10 times more frequent than the reactions to food additives identified in an earlier survey (*Young et al., 1987*). However, surveys which begin with questions based on public perceptions are subject to numerous errors, which Young attempted to minimize through interviews and challenge tests. The potential errors in surveys of this kind nevertheless merit further examination.

When attempting to assess the frequency of adverse reactions within a population, a number of constraints and difficulties arise. Kerr and colleagues (*1977*) designed a questionnaire which listed 18 food-associated symptoms, of which three (chest tightness, facial burning, numbness) were thought to be characteristically associated with the effects of monosodium glutamate. Using this questionnaire, he was able to identify possible cases of the 'Chinese Restaurant Syndrome' in 6.6% of those who replied. On receiving a second set of specific questions, including an enquiry as to whether they ate in Chinese restaurants and had heard of the adverse effects which can result, the same self-selected respondents gave answers suggesting that, in 31% of cases, there were adverse effects related to restaurant food.

Very different results were obtained, however, from a subsequent study which avoided the distortions which may arise with the use of leading questions. When two questionnaires which were designed to avoid bias were used (*Kerr et al., 1979*), the original figure of 6.6% with 'possible Chinese Restaurant Syndrome' dropped to 1.8%. Of this considerably smaller number, 2.3% (instead of 31%) were convinced that they had adverse effects related to restaurant food. Questionnaire-based prevalence studies are thus bedevilled by the problems of self-diagnosis, and by the added difficulty of making adequate allowance for those who do not respond to the questionnaire.

DO WE NEED THEM?

Although adverse reactions to food additives can occur, this does not justify the claim that these substances are responsible for a large number of illnesses in the general population, which could be avoided by a return to natural foods. At a time when food-transmitted infections are on the increase, and the number of illnesses and even deaths caused by gastroenteritis is rising, the removal of those additives which improve the keeping properties of food could have serious consequences. For every case in which there is a suspicion that an asthmatic or skin-whealing episode has been provoked by a food additive, there are several thousands of cases where adverse effects arise as a result of microbiological contamination of food.

There is no logical basis for an attack on food additives in general, as even the most traditional food processing involves the use of additives of one kind or another, whether the end product is a loaf of bread or a bottle of wine. Manufacturers have nevertheless responded to public pressure by offering the public a choice between foods which are conventionally processed and others which are advertised as containing no additives. Because these have a shorter shelf-life, foods that contain no additives may not only be expensive, but can be a potential cause of food-borne infection or illness caused by contamination with toxins. The problem, therefore, needs to be kept in perspective. It is reasonable to conclude that current procedures will continue to be necessary to monitor the safety of food additives. Where there are hazards involved in their use, the public should be kept informed.

For the general public, the permitted food additives have a substantial safety margin. However, for the benefit of those who wish to avoid these substances, and for the small number of susceptible people for whom particular additives may be harmful, it is important to provide informative labels as to the contents of processed foods, using the European numbering system as a convenient shorthand. This is the current requirement in most European countries. For those who are at risk, the British Ministry of Agriculture, Fisheries and Food produces a booklet, *Look At The Label*, which can be obtained by sending a request and a stamped self-addressed envelope to: FDIC, 25 Victoria Street, London, SW1H 0EX. Most of the major food supermarkets also provide nutritional advice in the form of publications on food additives and their uses.

In addition to detailed food-labelling, doctors and dieticians in the Netherlands, the United Kingdom and a few other countries now have access to databanks providing lists of food preparations which are free of certain foods or food additives known to cause adverse effects in susceptible individuals. The lists of food that are free of cow's milk, gluten or egg are those used most frequently, as these are the foods which cause the most problems. Food colours (E100–E180), sulphur dioxide (E220), sulphites (E221–227) and other preservatives (Table 7.2) are the additives most frequently suspected of causing adverse effects in susceptible individuals.

CONCLUSION

While it is understandable and, in some cases, desirable for the food industry to reduce the unnecessary additive content of food products, there is a need for more information from scientifically based studies rather than from the publicity of pressure groups, who are often mistaken in their attitudes and are often pursuing vested interests of their own. By following the advice of these agencies, many vulnerable people have been led to adopt diets which are inadequate and which are themselves the cause of disease. This applies particularly to those who attribute childhood behavioural disorders or hyperactivity to the effects of food additives or the food itself (see Chapter 2).

CHAPTER
—8—

Cow's Milk and Some Alternatives

As compared to human milk, cow's milk has a disproportionately high content of protein and other solutes, an unbalanced pattern of amino acids and, as far as the human baby is concerned, inadequate levels of essential fatty acids and nutrients, such as iron and zinc. However, even beyond infancy, milk remains a very important food. It not only provides protein, fat and water, but also contributes important nutrients to the diet. A two-year-old child can obtain all the calcium and riboflavin, half of the protein and a quarter of the recommended energy intake from 500 ml of cow's milk daily.

Unmodified cow's milk should not be used for infants below 6 months of age because the infant kidney cannot deal adequately with the high mineral content, and dehydration results. Because of the phosphate overload, there may also be a fall in serum calcium levels, in some cases leading to infantile fits, and there may be deficiencies of iron and vitamins C and D.

The British Department of Health (*DHSS, 1980*) has set guidelines which can help to approximate the composition of cow's milk-based formulas to that of human milk. Usually, the casein:whey ratio is altered, a mixture of vegetable and animal fats is used to boost the level of essential fatty acids and increase fat absorption, and supplements of iron and vitamin D are added. Nevertheless, these relatively simple modifications of cow's milk have caused gastrointestinal and other reactions sufficiently often to provide the stimulus for the establishment of large research programmes devoted to the design of better-tolerated cow's milk preparations.

It is not a new observation that cow's milk can cause health problems. Hippocrates observed, more than 2000 years ago, that it could cause both gastric upsets and a skin rash. Apart from the major role which cow's milk can play in the transmission of infection as well as the problem of lactose intolerance due to a deficiency of the enzyme lactase, up to 1% of infants in most communities are sensitive to cow's milk. The provoking factors which lead to sensitization have already been discussed, the most common being bottle-feeding, which may be followed by symptoms after a week to around 3 months after birth. Less frequently, the sensitizing protein comes from the mother during pregnancy and the child is sensitive at birth. Sensitization can also occur through breast-feeding when cow's milk protein taken by the mother may be present in her milk. The symptoms and diagnosis of allergy to cow's milk have been discussed in Chapter 6.

ALLERGENS OF COW'S MILK

The major allergens present in cow's milk (Table 8.1) are beta-lactoglobulin, alpha- and beta-casein, and alpha-lactalbumin. Allergy to immunoglobulin or lactalbumin is rare. Although beta-lactoglobulin accounts for only 10% of the total protein, it is a potent allergen for the human infant. The reasons are not clear, but it is the only type of

Table 8.1 Principal cow's milk proteins

Protein	Molecular weight	Quantity (mg/100 ml)	Percent of total protein
Caseins ($\alpha, \beta, \gamma, \varkappa$)	11,500–24,000	2500–2800	70–85
Albumin fractions	–	450–650	15–22
Beta-lactoglobulin	18,000–20,000	200–300	7–12
Alpha-lactalbumin	14,100	10–100	2–5
Serum albumin	66,500–69,000	30–40	0.1–1.3
Immunoglobulins	150,000–1,000,000	50–160	2–6

protein in cow's milk that is not present in human milk. Furthermore, it appears to resist acid digestion by the stomach so that undigested proteins are more likely to be presented to the intestinal epithelial cells.

The more severely affected cow's milk-allergic infants may have high blood levels of IgE antibodies to cow's milk proteins, but this is not an invariable finding. The evidence usually quoted concerning sensitization to the proteins of cow's milk is based on the detection of IgG antibodies in a baby's serum. This finding, however, shows no correlation with clinical evidence of cow's milk allergy (*Kemeny et al., 1991*) and may well indicate a normal response to proteins which have crossed the mucosal barrier. Almost all normal children and adults produce IgM and sometimes IgG antibodies to two or more cow's milk proteins, albeit at low levels. Children who are clinically sensitive to cow's milk usually react to several proteins, and high levels of IgG antibodies may be detected, especially to beta-lactoglobulin, but also to casein and bovine serum albumin. The circumstances which determine which molecules, or which parts of the molecule, stimulate the production of sensitized T cells and IgE antibody are the subject of current research.

ALTERNATIVES TO COW'S MILK

With the increased sophistication of food storage and distribution, milk products from goat and sheep, and even mozzarella cheese made from buffalo milk, have become available in many parts of the world. Infants who are intolerant of cow's milk may, however, develop sensitivities to any of these other milks, either immediately or after an interval.

In the United Kingdom, a relatively small number of around 3000 goatkeepers keep approximately 58,000 milking goats. Because there are fewer opportunities to bulk the milk with the yield from other herds, variations in composition can be striking, with fat percentages varying between 4–9% compared with less than 4% for cow's milk.

The whiteness of goat's milk and cheese is due to the absence of carotene, the precursor of vitamin A which gives cow's milk fat its yellow colour. Instead, goat's milk has a higher content of vitamin A itself, and is also lower in casein and polyunsaturated fatty acids than is cow's milk. An important difference between goat and human milk is, however, the high mineral load of the former (Table 8.2) with which, as with cow's milk, the infant kidney cannot deal satisfactorily. Goat's milk is also relatively rich in iron, but poor in vitamin C. For those who are highly sensitive to cow's milk, it should be noted that cow protein may be present in goat's milk products in the form of rennet used for coagulation.

Other alternatives to the use of cow's milk and its derivatives include mixtures which depend on chicken or beef protein reinforced with carbohydrate, fat, vitamins and minerals. By far the most commonly used, however, are soybean preparations. Soya milk is traditionally an aqueous extract of soybeans, or full-fat soybean flour, which has been heated to destroy the toxins which are present and then filtered. Soya-based formulas can cause fatty diarrhoea and a loss of minerals, vitamins and trace elements because of binding with the phytate they contain. They may also have a high aluminium content. These extracts tend to produce foul-smelling stools, and most soya milk infant formulas now use isolated soybean protein. They are also fortified with calcium, as their calcium content of 130 mg/l is insufficient for infant needs, and with methionine which, for the infant, is an important ingredient lacking in most soya preparations. Because feeding with soya has been associated with goitre in some cases, iodine is also added in addition to calcium and vitamins.

Soya preparations can have a useful, if limited, role. There is no convincing evidence to support their use in attempts to prevent the development of cow's milk allergy in babies whose parents have allergies and who are therefore at high risk of developing atopic disease. When a soya-based substitute was given instead of cow's milk to 232 infants with a family history of allergic disease, they fared slightly less

Table 8.2 Average mineral values for different types of milk

	Cow	Goat	Human
Sodium (mmol/l)	25	14	7
Potassium (mmol/l)	35	46	14
Calcium (mg/l)	1240	1280	340
Phosphorus (mg/l)	950	1049	140
Iron (mg/l)	1	5	1.5

(Modified from *Lawton*, 1984)

well than a matching control group, and half of them developed thrush. The soya preparations used may thus have an increased susceptibility to *Candida* infection (*Miskelly et al., 1988*).

Furthermore, 10–35% of infants who are given soya preparations because of cow's milk-protein intolerance develop soya-protein intolerance instead. This figure may, however, be inflated by the fact that some soya preparations appear to provoke diarrhoea because of their other components, including sucrose. Children with gastroenteritis have often been found to have persistent diarrhoea when treated with soya-protein mixtures. In a randomized study in which 40 children with gastroenteritis were given different soya preparations, it was shown that adverse reactions could be prevented by using lactose, instead of sucrose and dextromaltose, in the soya formula (*Donovan & Torres-Pinedo, 1987*).

COW'S MILK PROTEIN INTOLERANCE: PREVENTION, TREATMENT AND RESEARCH

The use of milk substitutes can provide an effective treatment for some infants who have already been sensitized, and controlled trials have shown that, for example, children with eczema benefit when cow's milk is excluded from their diet (*Atherton et al., 1978*). The more severe cases may also require injections of adrenaline and other resuscitative measures (see Chapter 6). It is not easy to predict, however, whether the use of an alternative diet will diminish or eliminate an infant's sensitivity to cow's milk. It is therefore important to focus research on methods of prevention and on modified forms of cow's milk which may be less allergenic.

Because of the increased risk of cow's milk allergy in infants born into atopic families, a great deal of attention has been focused on preventive measures in selected, high-risk cases. Dietary restrictions have been recommended for the mother during the last 3 months of pregnancy and during lactation, but with variable results. It is suggested that not only cow's milk, but also other major allergens – egg, chocolate and peanut – be eliminated from the maternal diet, and lactating mothers have been advised to eliminate dairy products and beef.

In spite of meticulous adherence to such dietary regimes, sensitization to cow's milk protein still occurs in some infants. For this reason, attention has been increasingly directed towards the possibility of manipulating infant feeds to diminish their allergenic effects. In an atopic child, it may be difficult to devise a modified form of cow's milk which achieves this aim and is yet acceptable to the child. Nevertheless, various types of processing have helped to achieve this, and efforts have also been made to link cow's milk protein to naturally occurring human proteins in an attempt to find a compound which does not stimulate the immune response. These last measures have been claimed to prevent the appearance of IgE antibodies in animals, provided that they have not already been sensitized. This is, however, far from applicable to a previously sensitized human subject.

The Case for Hydrolysates

Infant formulas based on hydrolysed milk proteins have been in clinical use for several decades. In the first few months of life, during which sensitization is most likely to occur, it is often claimed that a continuation of breast-feeding and a late introduction of cow's milk can reduce the incidence of food sensitization and eczema in children of allergic families. Cow's milk sensitization remains a problem, however, and attempts have therefore been made to alter the nature of the food allergens. As already noted, soya-protein preparations have been used extensively, in both the prevention and treatment of cow's milk-protein intolerance. These have, however, failed to prevent IgE-mediated disorders and, in babies already sensitized to cow's milk protein, have themselves led to reactions in many cases.

Infant formulas based on enzymatically produced protein hydrolysates have, in contrast, proved to be effective. In a few cases – perhaps 1–2% of those treated – infants who are already sensitized to cow's milk have continued to react to hydrolysates, possibly because some of the available preparations may contain too high a level of unhydrolysed protein. Although they do not all achieve the same level of safety, their place in the prevention of food allergy and atopic disorders in high-risk infants is now established.

Milk-formula feeds sometimes have several ingredients. Moneret-Vautrin and colleagues (1991) studied two infants with eczema who had been fed with a milk formula which was 10% vegetable lipids, 80% of which was peanut oil. When peanut oil was dropped inside the lower lip, both infants developed a generalized rash within 15 minutes. Skin-prick and RAST tests also gave positive results for peanut, but negative results for cow's milk allergy, and cow's milk was well tolerated thereafter. It is of interest that Taylor and co-workers (*1981*) and Keating and colleagues (*1990*) could detect no allergens in the peanut-oil preparations tested. The inclusion of these oils in milk formulas may nevertheless need to be reconsidered and their purity reassessed. Out of 45 preparations analysed in France, 11 contained peanut oil.

ALTERNATIVE APPROACHES TO MILK PROCESSING

Current processing methods include milk homogenization, pasteuriza-tion, sterilization by retorting or ultra-high-temperature heating (Table 8.3), and fermentation with lactic cultures. The effects of these different processes have been reviewed by Jost (*Jost et al., 1991*).

Milk Homogenization

The homogenization process aims to suppress creaming of the milk fat. This is achieved by reducing the size of the fat globules. This results in a large increase in fat surface and a migration of milk proteins (caseins and whey) to the surface of the fat globule. Because the charged protein molecules repel one another, these protein-coated small fat globules form a stable emulsion.

As with many other food processes, it has been suggested that milk homogenization has adverse effects. On theoretical grounds, it was suggested that a reduction in the size of fat globules could increase their absorption through the mucosal barrier and thereby increase their capacity to cause reactions. However, there is no evidence to support this theory. When 30 infants known to be allergic to cow's milk were tested with raw milk and pasteurized/homogenized milk, reactions were registered in 84% and 92% of the cases, respectively, a difference which was not statistically significant (*Hansen et al., 1987*). While there has been a suggestion that, in sensitized children, pasteurized/homogenized milk can sometimes produce more severe skin reactions than untreated milk, and that smaller quantities may be able to produce a clinical reaction (*Host & Samuelsson, 1988*), no major differences have, as yet, been demonstrated.

Effects of Heat-Processing

Guinea pigs are very susceptible to the effects of allergic reactions and have therefore been used in a number of studies in which milk processed in different ways is injected into these animals. In these studies, milk preparations which were strongly heated, such as sterilized liquid baby-formula preparations, appeared to be considerably less allergenic than pasteurized milk. Also, when extracts of milk were heated to 110–120°C for 10 minutes (retort treatment) and given to guinea pigs by mouth, the major proteins contained in whey (beta-lactoglobulin and alpha-lactalbumin) appeared to be harmless, although retort-treated casein still caused sensitization. This accords with the fact that whey proteins are complex in structure and easily denatured at temperatures above 70°C, whereas caseins are known to be remarkably heat-insensitive. The time taken for pasteurization and the temperature used (Table 8.3) is not likely to denature whey proteins, but denaturation occurs inevitably with retort sterilization. Ultra-high-temperature (UHT) heating takes an intermediate position.

Denaturation does not, in itself, produce milk which is free of

Table 8.3   Heat denaturation of milk whey protein in dairy processing

Process	Temperature	Holding time (sec)	Denaturation rate (%)[a]
Batch pasteurization	63–66°C	2000	3–10
HTST pasteurization	72–76°C	15–30	1–3
High pasteurization	80–90°C	4–15	1–10
UHT heating	130–140°C	2–15	30–70
Sterilization	110–120°C	1200–1800	> 99

UHT, ultra-high temperature; HTST, high temperature, short time.

([a] From *Dannenberg & Kessler, 1988*)

sensitizing properties, but species differences make it difficult to extrapolate the results of animal experiments to the human subject. Guinea pigs injected with denatured whey-protein preparations are as easily sensitized as with untreated milk. Denatured protein is more easily digested, however, and these findings cannot therefore be transposed to the effects of cow's milk taken by mouth in animals, let alone in humans. When the binding properties of IgE antibodies are studied in cow's milk-allergic individuals, it has been shown that heat treatment at 80–100°C for 15 minutes reduces the ability of beta-lactoglobulin and serum albumin to bind to the IgE, whereas little or no change is seen in alpha-lactalbumin and caseins. Heat denaturation may, therefore, reduce the allergenic capacity of some proteins but not others.

Because of the ease with which denatured proteins can be broken down by the digestive process, it may also be anticipated that some degree of protection will be provided by the intestinal tract. Nevertheless, heat-processing alone has failed to produce non-sensitizing milk preparations. It has even been claimed that, at high temperature, lactose can react with the protein present in milk (the Maillard reaction) and enhance its ability to provoke allergic reactions. Despite the ease with which IgG antibodies to these processed proteins can be raised in mice, there is no evidence that this has any relevance to the human subject.

Milk Fermentation and Cheese-Ripening

While the breakdown (proteolysis) of milk protein by fermentation can reduce its ability to cause allergic reactions, cheeses cannot be regarded as safe from this point of view, and fresh cheese or cheeses with a short ripening period are even less acceptable. During manufacture and ripening, a variety of enzymes break down the casein and whey proteins of the cheese mass. The amount of breakdown varies with the cheese, the local pH, and the salt content. The least breakdown occurs in the more peripheral parts of the cheese, where the salt concentration is highest but, in the low-salt zones, where breakdown of individual caseins can be very extensive, whey proteins are barely attacked at all.

In the manufacture of yoghurt, kefir and other fermented milks, a far less extensive breakdown is observed in the course of lactic fermentation with *Lactobacillus bulgaricus* or *Streptococcus thermophilus*.

Hyposensitizing Milk Formulas

One of the most stringent tests for 'hypoallergenic' milk preparations is based on whether they cause a reaction in previously sensitized individuals. In contrast to the disappointing results obtained with other methods, preparations containing protease-digested casein produce a very mild response in sensitive subjects, suggesting that the digestion of milk whey protein by protease may diminish its sensitizing capacity.

In this regard, the results of studies in guinea pigs have been of considerable value, and a reduced sensitizing capacity has been clearly demonstrated, especially after filtration to remove large (or undigested) fragments. The available clinical evidence has also been impressive. In one study of five children with immediate reactions to cow's milk, homogenized and pasteurized cow's milk produced positive skin-prick tests and demonstrably positive allergic reactions on oral challenge with milk quantities of between 5–75 ml. A casein hydrolysate preparation, on the other hand, did not elicit any reaction on skin-prick testing and produced no reaction on oral challenge with quantities exceeding 300 ml (*Host & Samuelsson, 1988*). Similarly encouraging results have been obtained by others.

Strategies for different types of proteolysis of milk proteins have therefore been developed, using enzymes which split the molecule at points where specific amino acids are placed. As the amino acids lysine and arginine are well distributed over the chain, cleaving at these sites by trypsin (obtained from porcine pancreas) results in well distributed cuts over the entire length of some major milk-protein molecules (*Jost et al., 1987*). While the larger fragments still appear to be allergenic, the smallest fragments are completely unreactive.

This has led to further studies in which whey protein has been digested by combining the effects of a specific protease, pepsin, with that of trypsin or chymotrypsin (*Asslin et al., 1989*). As a measure of the reduction in allergenic effect, binding of the whey protein fragments to IgE antibodies was assessed. All treatments inhibited binding to some extent, but the greatest reduction in binding was found when pepsin was used, followed by chymotrypsin.

These and similar studies have led to the clinical evaluation of a number of milk formulas prepared along these lines. A number of studies have been carried out in which formula-feeds have been given to babies at high risk of developing allergy; the results have shown that formula-feeds can produce a significantly lower incidence of allergic reactions than standard cow's milk or soya preparations. The benefit has been shown to continue throughout a 6-month feeding period and beyond. A study of high-risk infants (*Zeiger et al., 1989*) showed that, when given a casein hydrolysate as a supplement to breast milk, the cumulative prevalence of allergy was lower compared with that in infants given a standard infant milk formula consisting mainly of whey.

Another, less conclusive, study starts with the premise that infective gastroenteritis can predispose to the development of hypersensitive reactions to cow's milk protein (*Harrison et al. 1976*). The study involved the use of a protein hydrolysate formula (rather than cow's milk), which was given in the postinfective period to 23 infants who developed gastroenteritis before the age of 3 months. Two of the 23 developed cow's milk-protein hypersensitivity within 6 weeks of an *Escherichia coli* infection (*Hager et al., 1987*). Although this was not a controlled trial, it was suggested that the result compared favourably with earlier studies using similar methods, but feeding with cow's milk in the postinfective period (*Iyngkaran et al., 1979*).

In spite of the generally favourable results that have been reported, the use of protein hydrolysate formulas has its problems. First, they can be very expensive. Comparisons between old and newer preparations have yet to be carried out, and the unpleasant taste of several of the preparations has not been satisfactorily overcome. There is, nevertheless, encouraging evidence that protease-treated formulas may be helpful in infants who already have a clinically manifest milk intolerance. Although there have been some cases reported where proteolysed products of both casein and whey have caused anaphylactic reactions in previously sensitized subjects, this may be an indication of the presence of low amounts of unchanged peptide or protein that are still detectable using highly sensitive techniques. It remains to be considered whether it is ethical and possible to use the response of sensitized individuals as a continuing means of testing the adequacy of individual preparations of casein or whey treated by proteolysis.

Even if appropriate formula-feeds can be developed at an acceptable cost, it should be noted that their safety will depend on their handling during reconstitution. This depends, as much as anything else, on the availability of drinking water for this purpose that is safe bacteriologically and uncontaminated by nitrates or lead. Softened water should not be used because of its high sodium content, and the feeds must be accurately reconstituted with due attention to sterility.

CONCLUSION

Unmodified cow's milk contains too much sodium and phosphate for the infant kidney to deal with. It is also too rich in protein and too poor in essential fatty acids. Although simple modifications can improve the mixture, adverse reactions can be caused by both modified and unmodified cow's milk. Large-scale research programmes have, therefore, aimed at finding alternatives or developing better tolerated preparations.

Although alternatives to cow's milk can be of value, those based on goat's or sheep's milk, or soya, all have disadvantages. Fermented milk products are sometimes better tolerated than milk itself, but the difference may not be substantial. Heat denaturation also has a limited positive effect.

The breakdown of milk proteins by enzymes (pepsin and trypsin or chymotrypsin) may be of value in sensitized infants. Proteolysed preparations are therefore increasingly used, but the degree of proteolysis – and therefore the degree of safety – varies in different preparations. To be safe, they must also be carefully reconstituted, and their expense and unpleasant taste are disadvantages which have yet to be overcome.

CHAPTER
—9—

Gluten Sensitivity and Coeliac Disease

Coeliac disease is an illness that is most likely to appear in early childhood after the introduction of cereal foods to the diet. Most child coeliacs are diagnosed before the age of 2 years. The classical description is that of a child who fails to thrive, has striking fatty diarrhoea, an enlarged abdomen, limp muscles, weakness and a bad temper.

The tendency to develop the disease appears to be inherited, and a convenient definition is that coeliac disease is a genetically determined disease in which there is an abnormal reaction to some of the storage proteins (prolamins) in wheat, rye, barley and oats which damages the small intestinal wall, thus interfering with absorption of all nutrients in the affected part of the intestine.

The relationship to diet was first described by Samuel Gee (1888) who noted that, in the '. . . coeliac affection . . . the allowance of farinaceous food must be small: highly starched food, rice, sago, corn-flour are unfit . . . If the patient can be cured at all,' wrote Gee, 'it must be by means of diet.' This theme was developed by others; Parsons (1932) recognized that coeliac disease did not occur in infants who were still being breast-fed, and Sheldon (1949) observed that fatty diarrhoea was much reduced when foods containing flour were excluded. The significance of these observations was dramatically demonstrated by Dicke (1950), a Dutch paediatrician who had noted, during World War II, that a wartime diet of mostly potatoes, tulip bulbs and cabbage was of benefit to those diagnosed as having coeliac diarrhoea, while most other children in his care lost weight. Starting from this point, and from a number of previous observations on the harmful effects of biscuits, bread and flour-containing meals, Dicke and his colleagues (*van der Kamer et al., 1953*) made a number of further advances. They showed that gluten and, in particular, one of its components, gliadin, was the toxic factor in wheat that caused damage to the intestinal wall of children with coeliac disease. They found a similar factor in the storage proteins from rye, oats and barley, and recommended that wheat, barley, oats and rye be excluded from the diet.

COELIAC DISEASE AND PROLAMIN TOXICITY

The search for the damaging aspect of the molecule has taken much longer, but considerable efforts continue to be made to obtain accurate information as to its nature. The reason is a very practical one. It is a relatively simple matter to set up an assay system for testing foods to ensure that they are gluten-free. If the toxic part of the molecule were fully identified, it might then be possible to identify a further range of foods, or even a type of wheat, that contained storage proteins but lacked the toxic component. This goal has yet to be achieved.

Cereals of the Gramineae family are the most widely grown crops in the world and the most important source of protein for human nutrition. There is a close genetic relationship between wheat and rye, followed by barley and oats and, more distantly, rice and maize. This is reflected in the similarity of the storage proteins in general and, in particular, the prolamins of these cereals. The storage proteins have no special function within the grain other than to provide a store of nutrients and energy, and consist of albumins, globulins and prolamins of different types. The prolamins have been the most studied.

Prolamins provide a store of nitrogen for the germinating plant. Around 40% of the amino-acid residues are glutamine and approximately 17% are proline. Although the similarity between the prolamines of closely related cereals is not apparent from their names (Table 9.1), they are sufficiently alike to provoke an immunological response in humans that shows considerable cross-reactivity between

Table 9.1 Protein and prolamin content of the cereal grains

Cereal	Protein content (%)	Prolamin type	Prolamin content (%)
Wheat	10–15	Gliadin	4–7.5
Rye	9–14	Secalin	3–7
Barley	10–14	Hordein	3.5–7
Oats	8–14	Avenin	0.8–2.1
Maize	7–13	Zein	3.5–7

one prolamin and another. Such cross-reactivity is much less for cereals of other subfamilies.

The prolamin of wheat is gluten, which can be further separated into glutemin and gliadin. From around the age of 3 years, the gliadin intake does not normally fall below approximately 2 g daily. In a young adult, it may be four times as much. When the proteins of wheat flour are eliminated by washing, a wheat starch is obtained with a low protein content, consisting mainly of gluten and a starch granule (non-prolamin) protein. When the protein content of wheat starch is reduced to below 0.25%, the gliadin content is reduced to zero (Fig. 9.1). Such observations have helped to delineate the requirements for wheat-starch preparation to render it safe for coeliac patients to ingest.

It has now been concluded that alpha-gliadin is toxic to coeliac patients, and several toxic fragments have been identified after digestion with trypsin. Many proteins in the gliadin mixture, however, share the same peptides in their structure. Attempts to identify the possible toxic sequences in gliadin have been vigorously pursued, but attempts to test their ability to cause damage to the intestinal cells of coeliac disease patients have met with ethical difficulties when it comes to testing their effects upon patients. A number of small proteins have been synthesized to replicate part of the gliadin molecule, but none has been found to damage either human intestinal cells grown in culture medium or rat intestine. The decisive test, therefore, requires that the suspect substance be administered to patients who have recovered from coeliac disease and shown, by means of serial intestinal samples, to cause damage to the intestinal mucosa. Work of this kind has been limited, but it has been shown that an 18,000 MW peptide fragment isolated from a trypsin digest of alpha-gliadin can still cause intestinal damage in susceptible patients.

The next research target after the identification of the toxic

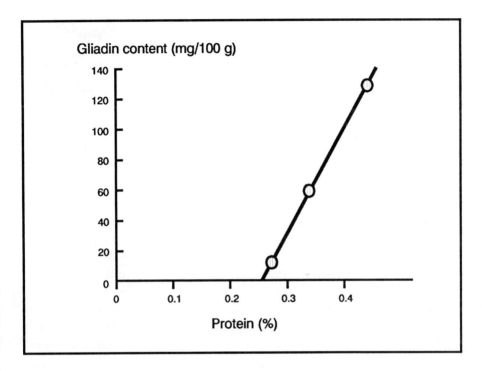

Fig. 9.1
Relationship between gliadin and protein nitrogen content of wheat starches. This provides the basis of processing foods that are safe for coeliac patients. Courtesy of Hekkens, 1991.

sequence of gliadin will be the production of highly specific, artificially produced (monoclonal) antibodies to that sequence. As in other situations, these antibodies could be used as highly specific chemical reagents in the analysis of gluten-free food. Biotechnological manipulations of the amino-acid sequence of gluten within the wheat germ may also be possible and thus help in the development of crops containing non-toxic prolamin.

NATURE OF GLUTEN SENSITIVITY

There is still no agreement as to whether coeliac disease is caused by an enzyme deficiency, an immune disorder, an adhesive (lectin-like) action which causes direct damage, or a membrane defect. Patients with active coeliac disease appear to lack important enzymes in the lining cells of the intestine. As the loss of brush-border enzymes is not uncommon in other forms of intestinal disease (*Haffejee, 1991*), some of this enzyme loss may be a mere consequence of intestinal damage. With a gluten-free diet, nearly all enzymes have been shown to revert to a normal level, but deficiencies of transglutaminase and angiotensin-converting enzyme may persist, suggesting that not all of the enzyme loss is due to this cause.

The theory of an immune disturbance has come closer to explaining the changes seen in coeliac disease, especially as a gluten challenge leads rapidly to the presence, in the intestinal mucosa, of the type of T cell known to cause tissue destruction. It is clear, however, that many of the immunological changes thought to explain the cause of the disease are, in fact, secondary phenomena. The blood levels of antigliadin IgA and IgG antibodies is much higher in coeliac patients than in control subjects, but these levels return to normal with a gluten-free diet, despite the fact that the susceptibility to gluten damage persists. Similar antibodies are also found in the blood of patients who have other forms of food sensitivity, such as egg allergy (*Kemeny et al., 1986*), suggesting that these antibodies represent a reaction to any food protein which crosses a damaged mucosal membrane. Despite the convincing nature of the T-cell infiltration seen in coeliac disease, it remains possible that their appearance is secondary to some other process rather than the prime cause of the disease.

More recent antibody studies have raised further possibilities concerning the part played by immune reactions in coeliac disease. Antibodies have been identified that react with different components of human intestinal tissue and may therefore be regarded as autoantibodies. Antireticulin antibodies have been recognized for some years by means of a fluorescent test. In essence, this test depends on the staining pattern, in the form of a network (reticulum), achieved after a patient's serum has been added to a section of intestinal tissue on a microscope slide. Their presence correlates well with the presence of coeliac disease, but not as well as do antibodies which bind to endomysium (EMA), the sheath which surrounds the smooth muscle cells and bundles.

Anti-EMA antibodies of the IgA class correlate with the severity of the mucous-membrane lesion and disappear after gluten withdrawal (*Anon, 1991*). Human non-collagen protein molecules have now been identified which may be the tissue components against which both the antireticulin and anti-EMA antibodies are directed (*Maki et al., 1991*). As there is no cross-reaction between these antibodies and gliadin, they may represent a true autoimmune response, but their role in the disease process is still obscure.

Other theories concerning the origin of coeliac disease are more speculative. It has been suggested that gliadin initiates cell damage because it sticks to the intestinal cell membrane in coeliac patients, but not in normal controls. However, although 'adhesion molecules' can be produced (*Sturgess et al., 1990*), attempts to show that they can bind to live tissue have not succeeded. Similarly, there is no evidence of a primary defect in the structure of the cell membrane that increases membrane permeability and thus allows the increased penetration of proteins. This also remains an unsupported theory.

As the villous atrophy of coeliac disease – and the circulating antibodies with which it is associated – can develop in previously normal subjects, it follows that an inherited susceptibility cannot be the only factor involved. In such cases, it has been suggested (*Lancet, 1991*) that an added factor is required, such as a coincident adenovirus infection. In keeping with this is the evidence quoted in Chapter 6, suggesting that other types of food-induced villous atrophy can be triggered by an intestinal infection. It is even possible that other types of villous damage – for example, caused by cow's milk – can set the scene for the subsequent development of gluten intolerance (*Gryboski et al., 1965*). In those with an inherited susceptibility to gluten enteropathy (in contrast to those with mucosal damage caused by other foods), the sensitivity to gluten and its ability to cause mucosal damage tend to persist indefinitely, once they have been established.

Racial and Geographical Prevalence

Coeliac disease has been most studied in Western Europe and is said to be related to the cereal-eating habits of these countries. The prevalence in Ireland may be as high as one in 303 (*Mylotte et al., 1973*). The prevalence in Austria is similar to that in the Galway area of Ireland, suggesting that genetic factors may operate. Tissue-typing studies have confirmed this. The tissue types A1, B8, DR3 and DPw1, which are most closely associated with the disease (*Hall et al., 1991*), are nevertheless shared by many unaffected people. In addition, the prevalence in North America is much lower than in Europe among people of the same ethnic origins, supporting the view that factors other than genetic must influence the development of the disease. In England and Scotland, the prevalence has been calculated to be between one in 1100 and one in 4000, respectively, and the rates in Sweden, Switzerland, Norway, France and The Netherlands are somewhat similar to that in the United Kingdom.

Coeliac disease is known to occur in Brazil, Argentina, South Africa and Australasia, and the observation that this has been diagnosed in those of European stock (*Cooke & Holmes, 1983*) has been taken to emphasize the importance of a genetic factor. However, coeliac disease is also found in Indians, Cubans, Mexicans, Arabs and in those of Arab-African stock. Diet may well provide an additional factor, and the increased incidence of coeliac disease during the 1950s and 1960s may have been provoked by the practice of introducing cereals into an infant's diet very early on, often at the age of only 4–6 weeks. It has been suggested that the apparent decrease since 1974 may have followed the reversal of this practice. While there is no proof that diet is a determining factor, it should be noted that, in India, coeliac disease is found in the wheat-eating areas of Bengal and the Punjab, and not in the rice-eating areas of Southern India. It is possible that the type of wheat grown may also be important, as the toxic component may not occur to the same extent in different varieties (*Ciclitira et al., 1980*).

Clinical Features

The classical presentation of coeliac disease in early childhood is with diarrhoea, weakness and a 'pot belly' in an ill and fretful child. In even younger children, there may be a tendency to vomit after feeding, and loss of appetite is a prominent symptom whereas the older children usually eat normally. A very early onset may be accompanied by such severe weakness that there is an inability to walk or even stand. Severe malnutrition and swelling of the legs due to protein deficiency may be in evidence, together with a failure to gain weight. In older children, growth retardation may be the most prominent or, sometimes, the only clinical symptoms. A number of less severe cases undoubtedly remain undiagnosed, presenting in adult life or even in elderly men or women who develop a malignant change and present with a lymphoma (*Jansen et al., 1991*).

The ratio of women to men has been estimated to be around 1.26:1 (*Cooke & Holmes, 1983*). In addition to the patients who present in childhood, there is also a peak incidence in women in the fourth decade, and in the sixth and seventh decades in men (*Swinson & Levi, 1980*).

The late diagnosis of the milder cases of coeliac disease may sometimes occur because they are totally symptomless, or because of the lack of simple diagnostic screening tests. For years, the measurement of faecal fat provided the sole cumbersome technique for establishing the presence of fatty diarrhoea, which was the only screening test available and, being crude, gave a positive result in most cases. However, when the characteristic damage to the villi of the intestine was described (Fig. 9.2), and it became possible to sample the cells lining the intestine, the demonstration of these changes became the chief diagnostic requirement. Many more cases were then discovered, sometimes associated with other disorders, such as diabetes mellitus, Down's syndrome or IgA deficiency.

More recently, there has been a search for non-invasive test methods. As noted above, the presence of specific antigliadin antibodies is now used as a screening test and, although it may represent a secondary consequence of the condition, tests which confine their attention to antigliadin antibodies of the IgA class have been claimed to show a high degree of specificity (*McMillan et al., 1991*) and may be of considerable value in selecting patients for further investigation. The autoantibodies, which have also been mentioned above, include antireticulin and anti-EMA antibodies, and also provide reasonably specific indicators of the jejunal damage seen in coeliac disease (*Lancet, 1991*). As they disappear when gluten is withdrawn from the diet, these autoantibodies may be yet another example of a reaction to the disease rather than the cause. Their value in preliminary diagnosis may, however, be considerable; they appear to be markers of a latent form of the disease, as their presence can precede jejunal damage in the relatives of coeliac patients who later develop the disease (*Maki et al., 1991*). In general, those antibodies which disappear on a gluten-free diet are equally likely to reappear with the reintroduction of gluten. There are, however, occasional patients who lose both their gluten sensitivity and their antigliadin antibodies on a gluten-free diet and who show no subsequent increase in antigliadin antibody after a gluten challenge. The more specific antibody tests which have now been introduced may

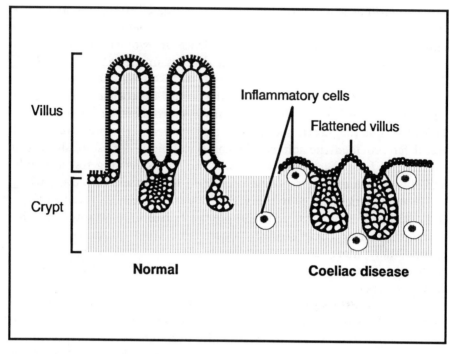

Fig. 9.2

The characteristic loss of intestinal absorptive surfaces is now diagnostic of coeliac disease. The normal finger-like villi and their hair-like microvilli provide a large absorptive surface (left); in coeliac disease, the villi are flattened and there is enlargement of the crypts.

make it easier to follow the progress of such patients in the future and to assess whether their gluten sensitivity has disappeared.

Unusual Presentations

It is usually the younger patients who present with severe illness, but there are others who remain virtually symptomless or have only non-specific complaints; in such cases, the diagnosis may be difficult, but not impossible. The diagnosis will depend on an increased awareness of the significance of minor biochemical abnormalities or haematological changes. These changes may amount to no more than a hypochromic anaemia, or the appearance of the so-called Howell-Jolly bodies, which are dark spots within the red blood cells. As such malformed cells are normally removed by the spleen, their presence in the circulating blood may point to the presence of splenic atrophy, a condition closely associated with coeliac disease. Other changes that may reflect poor function of the spleen are an increased number of blood platelets and the finding of other types of deformed red cells carrying such descriptive names as target cells, burr cells and acanthocytes.

It should be noted that the splenic atrophy of coeliac disease is accompanied by a generalized reduction in lymphatic tissue which is not affected by treatment with a gluten-free diet (*Trewby et al., 1981*). The hypochromic anaemia of coeliac disease has already been mentioned. Iron deficiency contributes to this anaemia, both because of poor absorption through the damaged mucous membrane, and because of an increased excretion of iron into the gut (*Kosnai et al., 1979*). The size of the red cells may also increase (macrocytosis) because of poor absorption of folic acid. Folic-acid deficiency is also responsible for some abnormalities in the mucous membrane, such as shortening of the villi, increased crypt length and enlargement of the nuclei in the mucosal cells (*Davidson & Townley, 1977*). The changes due to iron and folate deficiencies are corrected by withdrawing gluten from the diet.

Apart from the symptoms of malaise, nausea, loss of appetite, abdominal distention, looseness of stool and, in some cases, vomiting and abdominal pain, coeliac disease may also present with some less characteristic features which are not easily recognized. Although not true of all patients, short stature is a common feature, although normal growth is restored when gluten is excluded from the diet. Puberty may be delayed, and menstrual disturbances and diminished fertility are common in older women (*Ferguson et al., 1982*). Again, a gluten-free diet may restore normal function relatively rapidly. There also appears to be an association with ulcers in the mouth (aphthous stomatitis), which may precede other manifestations of coeliac disease by many years and disappear when a gluten-free diet is introduced. More dramatically, patients may experience 'gluten shock', a condition first described by van der Kamer and co-workers (*1953*) as an abnormally violent reaction to even a small amount of food containing wheat. Such episodes occurred within 3–6 hours of ingestion, and involved severe abdominal pain, vomiting, pallor and sometimes a state of shock.

Mood changes are common in patients with coeliac disease, both treated and untreated. The diet itself requires an attention to detail which many patients find difficult. In one large series of cases (*Cooke & Holmes, 1983*), 31 out of 314 proven cases of coeliac disease needed treatment for depression. Organic dementia and schizophrenia have also been described. The prevalence of schizophrenia has been estimated at between 10–37/1000 coeliac patients compared with 2.3–4.7/1000 in the general population. Although this association has been disputed (*Selmer & Staudenmayer, 1991*), it has been claimed that the mental changes appear to be arrested on withdrawal of gluten from the diet (*Cooke, 1976*). It has been suggested that impaired hydroxylation of tyrosine in the synthesis of amine transmitters, such as dopamine, noradrenaline and adrenaline, may play a part in causing these effects (*Leeming & Blair, 1980*), or that gluten-derived peptides, shown to be deposited in brain tissue, may have a toxic effect (*Zioudrou et al., 1979*).

Mucosal Damage and its Effect on Symptoms

Not all gluten intolerance is associated with mucosal damage, and 'non-coeliac' cases have been described in which there is gluten-sensitive diarrhoea, but with a normal appearance of the intestinal lining (*Cooper et al., 1980*). In coeliac disease itself, mucosal damage is mainly seen in the upper small intestine, and its effects include a reduced synthesis of mucosal enzymes, such as disaccharidases and peptidases, and a reduced production of intestinal hormones. There is also a change towards alkalinity of the intestinal contents (*Lucas et al., 1978*), which may so impair the absorption of drugs and nutrients that, in the long term, deficiency states are likely to occur. The lack of mucosal enzymes not infrequently results in lactose intolerance, which is itself a cause of diarrhoea and irritable bowel symptoms. There is also an active secretion of sodium in the upper jejunum of the coeliac patient that cannot always be compensated by an increased absorption of water and electrolytes in the distal small bowel. As a result of diarrhoea, there is an increased loss of potassium, and there may also be a loss of zinc and magnesium. Those who have severe electrolyte loss may develop lethargy and weakness, irritability, confusion, forgetfulness, muscle spasms, poor coordination, fits, loss of taste and infertility. Electrolyte disturbances, if uncorrected, can also lead to renal tubular damage and increased urinary excretion at night. In untreated cases, absorption of vitamin D is usually impaired and, because of the excess of fat in the stool, calcium absorption may also be reduced. The muscle weakness of vitamin D deficiency is an occasional early symptom, and the soft bones of osteomalacia are commonly seen. In addition, there is the loss of bone matrix as seen in osteoporosis. These abnormalities are reversed by withdrawing gluten, but even without gluten withdrawal, calciferol by mouth nearly always cures the osteomalacia (*Cooke & Holmes, 1983*).

Less common changes associated with coeliac disease include peripheral nerve lesions which remain unexplained, as they are not helped by a gluten-free diet and are unrelated to either folic acid or vitamin B_{12} deficiency. In 5–8% of patients who were followed for more than 10 years, numbness, tingling, pain, weakness and an unsteady gait were noted, and changes in the central nervous system may also occur, for example, atrophic changes in the brain and cerebellum together with patchy lesions in the spinal cord which are distinct from the lesions seen in vitamin B_{12} deficiency.

It is also well recognized that, in longstanding coeliac disease, there is an increased incidence of malignant disease, including T-cell lymphoma and carcinoma, especially in the intestinal tract. Patients who fail to respond to a gluten-free diet, or who deteriorate after a period of good health, may lose weight, or develop abdominal pain and diarrhoea which cannot be explained without further investigation to exclude a malignant lymphoma. A gluten-free diet diminishes the risk of a T-cell intestinal lymphoma in patients with coeliac disease (*Holmes et al., 1989*), and this has been used as an indication for continuing a gluten-free diet for life, even though its abandonment may lead to no obvious evidence of relapse.

One last association with coeliac disease is provided by dermatitis herpetiformis, a symmetrical rash on the knees, elbows, buttocks, face and trunk, which sometimes includes lesions within the mouth. The rash consists of small papules and vesicles which may be very scanty at any given time. When the intestinal mucosa is biopsied, around 25% of cases show mucosal damage identical to that found in untreated coeliac disease. Approximately 50% of patients show less severe changes. The remainder show apparently normal appearances except for slightly increased numbers of lymphocytes in the epithelium. Frank symptoms of coeliac disease are unusual in these cases, and the rash is improved in over 90% of patients by a gluten-free diet, regardless of the appearances of the intestinal mucosa (*Reunala et al., 1977*).

DIETARY MANAGEMENT

Whatever the clinical presentation of coeliac disease, the only treatment remains the gluten-free diet. As gluten is used in numerous thickeners, emulsifiers and substitutes for animal protein, this is not an easy task. The standard for gluten-free wheat flour stipulated by the Codex Alimentarius Committee implies a gliadin content of around 30 mg/ 100 g of wheat flour, although a working group on prolamin toxicity has proposed a level of 10 mg of gliadin/100 g of cereal flour as the uppermost limit for a food to be called gluten-free. In analysing the gliadin content of food, several methods have been developed, especially those using monoclonal antibodies.

A child with coeliac disease who has lost mucosal intestinal cells may also have to contend with the loss of enzymes, such as lactase. For this reason, when a gluten-free diet is introduced, it may first be necessary to restrict lactose. In severely malnourished children, long-chain fats are also poorly absorbed, and a dietitian's help will ensure that the type of fat eaten is appropriately changed. During this phase, the use of protein hydrolysates may also be helpful although, after the first 3 months, restriction of gluten is all that is necessary.

By the age of adolescence, the discipline required with a gluten-free diet may be difficult to follow. However, it is not necessarily the case that the less conscientious children will experience symptoms at this age, and it is therefore difficult to be certain whether the liberties taken with the diet can put patients more at risk of developing late complications. Although one such complication may be the late development of gastrointestinal cancer (*Holmes et al., 1989*), their long-term prospects have yet to be fully assessed.

CONCLUSION

Coeliac disease can present in a wide variety of ways and, although the majority of cases are diagnosed in early childhood, a substantial number come to light only in later life. Despite the occasional patient in whom the sensitivity to gluten may disappear completely, the only treatment which can be generally recommended is the long-term maintenance of a gluten-free diet.

CONCLUSION

In considering the ways in which the management of coeliac disease may yet be improved, attempts are being made to modify or degrade gluten, and to develop wheat variants which do not contain the toxic peptide. As genetic factors are undoubtedly involved, there is also the possibility that, in future, there may be the possibility of identifying and manipulating the relevant genes.

CHAPTER
—10—

The Patient's Dilemma

For the majority of people who develop food reactions, the one or two foods which cause problems are relatively easily identified and avoided. However, the most alarming reactions are those involving the immediate type of allergy, making it necessary to inquire into the contents of, for example, sauces and salad dressings, the method of cooking, or the ingredients in cakes and cooked dishes, with a small number of ingredients in mind. Usually, this is likely to include fish or shellfish, egg, nuts or milk, although wheat, soya, sesame seeds, grape products (including wine vinegar), spices (including mustard) and the foods listed in Table 6.4 can present problems in some cases.

The patient who has to cope with an insidious, but less immediate, form of food reaction is much more likely to encounter difficulties. The first arises because of the available, somewhat limited, methods of diagnosis and the scepticism that is often aroused in doctors, dietitians, and even friends and acquaintances. A careful enquiry into the content of cooked dishes may nevertheless be necessary if clinical reactions to food are to be avoided when a meal is taken away from home. Restaurant foods may also be contaminated with materials from a cooking utensil or another customer's dish, which an individual cannot easily identify, but may cause problems for highly susceptible individuals.

The mother of a food-allergic child is likely to encounter even more difficult problems, especially when the child is at school or visiting friends, environments in which some protection is needed, but without placing too much emphasis on the child's disability. For the benefit of mothers of allergic children in general, or of children with coeliac disease, asthma or eczema, the development of patient self-help groups has been of great benefit.

INITIATING A DIET

The institution of a food-elimination diet carries risks as well as benefits, and should always be preceded by the diagnostic procedures outlined in Chapter 6. When grossly restricted diets are prescribed on the basis of an imperfect history, combined with such unreliable test methods as cytotoxic or immune-complex tests, neutralization tests or sublingual tests, there is the danger − almost an inevitability − that a prolonged course of dietary treatment is initiated before a valid diagnosis has been made. The risks of malnutrition or the neglect of an associated disease have already been mentioned, and other examples have been published (*Bierman et al., 1978; Lloyd-Still, 1979; David et al., 1984; Robertson et al., 1988; Labib et al., 1989; Condemi, 1991*). In addition, elimination diets can themselves impose a considerable emotional and physical strain on an entire family. There can be major difficulties over the purchase and preparation of meals, and the social isolation − which can be a genuine hazard − when meals cannot easily be eaten away from home. If a diagnosis of food allergy is made on inadequate grounds, it often reinforces an unjustified parental obsession with diet. The physician may then be involved in reinforcing a parent's fanciful notions which, at their extreme, lead to the dietary rigidity or other measures characteristic of the form of child abuse known as Munchausen's disease by proxy (see Chapter 6).

Assessing a patient's nutritional state and requirements is, ideally, the province of the dietitian, who can also assess the vitamin and mineral requirements in comparison to the recommended dietary allowances (RDAs) established by the American National Academy of Sciences. The caloric and protein requirements of children depend on their age and, except in the obese, on their weight (Table 10.1). The

Table 10.1 Caloric and protein requirements in children

Age of child (years)	Daily kcal/kg	Daily protein (g/kg)
Less than 1	100–110	1.6–2.2
1–3	100	1.2
4–10	70–90	1.0–1.1
Preadolescents and adolescents	40–55	0.8–1.0

(Koerner & Sampson, 1991)

protein, if not of animal origin, should be of sufficiently good quality to provide all the essential amino acids (*Koerner & Sampson, 1991*), and the carbohydrates should emphasize the more complex and starchy substances rather than the simple sugars. As animal fats are of the saturated variety, at least some unsaturated fat should be provided in the form of vegetable oils and margarines.

The choice of foods should consider quality as well as quantity. Protein of high biological value is found in egg, milk products, poultry, meat or fish, but those on vegan diets, which exclude animal foods, may need advice on an appropriate mixture of the vegetable proteins that can provide adequate quantities of essential amino acids. This may require a full record of the dietary intake for a period of up to a week and the help of a dietitian in providing a dietary analysis. If the diet is inadequate, supplements of vitamins, minerals or other deficient substances should be given. In addition, in the case of a child, a regular check should be kept on height and weight for comparison with standard national tables to detect any evidence of stunting or wasting.

PATIENT SELF-HELP GROUPS

An excellent example of a food reaction that should be tackled with care and persistence is the problem of coeliac disease. Coeliac societies have now been established in a large number of countries, mostly through the enthusiasm of non-medical people who have a personal or familial involvement with coeliac disease. Having discovered how difficult it may be to get good advice on dietary matters, many public-spirited people have contributed by providing leaflets, booklets and personal advice to patients who have this condition and, as the self-help movement has grown, for a widening range of other chronic diseases. As an example, a Dutch food-allergy association (NVAS) has been established by Nieborg-Eshuis, and has its own Medical Board of Advisers, produces a quarterly publication, and has invited comments from advocates of alternative medicine for consideration by its Board. Its 35 support groups meet regularly, and their efforts extend to a telephone-enquiry service and a dietary-advice group. In collaboration with the Dutch Education Bureau of Food and Nutrition, this organization has established a food-intolerance databank, so that information on the constituents of commercially prepared foods can be made available to all patients who are intolerant to certain foods. Similar databanks have been established in Great Britain and other countries so that dietitians and others can have easy access to such information.

A further initiative has been taken by various governments, notably in the European Community, who have required food-labelling of commercial products. This has been of the greatest help to those who have to face the practical difficulties of keeping to a rigorous diet. Ambivalent attitudes have developed, however, to the E numbers which provide a shorthand for manufacturers to identify the food additives that have been tested by the European Community and regarded as safe. The survey which listed the components of spinach and drew attention to the E numbers within this food brought a simple response from most of the housewives questioned – that they would not knowingly buy a food containing those components.

The dietary problems of food-allergic children are particularly difficult, as these children may also have other allergy-related problems as well as having associated allergies to household dust and pets, grass pollen or flowers. In severe cases, before a child visits friends or goes to a party, the parents will have to telephone the hosts and ask if the visitor may bring special foods. The child who appears healthy, but has to restrict a valuable food such as milk, may not be able to convince members of the family that such measures are necessary, and the parent who has to offer repeated explanations may feel despondent and isolated, not only within the community, but within the family itself. There may be difficulties, for example with a grandparent who sees such restrictions as a withdrawal of parental love, for which the grandparent takes the responsibility of providing a substitute!

It is a common perception, within self-help groups, that the presence of asthma or eczema helps to persuade others of the need for special care. The presence of hidden handicaps in apparently healthy children may make the condition more difficult to accept as far as the general public is concerned. From the medical viewpoint, this must arouse considerable sympathy, but also a particular concern over the basis on which a diagnosis is made. Children with coeliac disease may indeed have a hidden handicap, but self-help groups which give uncritical support to the use of restrictive diets for hyperactive children should be advised of the dangers which may arise from misdiagnosis.

MATERNAL PROBLEMS

The mother who is aware of allergic problems within the family may have to anticipate likely problems before they occur. It is difficult to ban pets from the home of a child who has already become fond of the pet but has developed an allergic reaction. It is equally difficult to restrict a child's diet once a food allergy has developed. Although she may not always succeed, the mother who stops smoking during pregnancy, avoids having pets in the house, follows the preventive dietary measures in pregnancy (as detailed in Chapter 6), and breast-feeds her baby will have done all that is, at present, possible to prevent the development of allergies in her child. If her child nevertheless develops an allergy to a food, the problem has to be faced by the entire family, especially when the child is not old enough to take independent action.

The mother who has to arrange dietary measures for a child with coeliac disease, or who is allergic to cow's milk or egg, may have to consider whether error is best avoided by restricting the diet of the rest of the family along with the patient. The child who must become accustomed to confronting the forbidden foods when outside of the home may have to learn that other members of the family are allowed foods which the child must nevertheless regard as prohibited. Undoubtedly, there are problems when a child is asked to cooperate with unpopular measures, or refuse sweets while away from home – unless perhaps the forbidden sweet can be replaced by one from the child's own supply. In younger children, it is difficult to devise ways to prevent the child from stealing prohibited food that can be damaging or dangerous.

One of the problems of all special diets is their cost, for which solutions may be available in some countries, but not in others. The problem may not easily be solved where protein hydrolysates or other expensive foods are needed, and help may be needed both from dietitians and from patient self-help groups, which can usually provide information on the resources available through health insurance, the National Health Service in general, and Social Security funds.

A mother's problems in shopping may also require the help of support groups, who can sometimes provide important practical information on foods that are available only in particular supermarkets or shops. Help can also be obtained from a databank list of manufactured foods which are, for example, gluten- or egg-free. With such restrictions, however, there is a great need for the professional advice of the dietitian to avoid deficiencies of calcium and vitamins. There is a need to emphasize the necessity for professional supervision of unusual or restricted diets of any kind.

DIETARY ERRORS

Most children adapt surprisingly well to a diet, however strict it may be. Even the greatest care, however, cannot always prevent the inadvertent exposure to an allergenic food. When Bock and Atkins (1989) followed-up children who had severe peanut allergy, 16 out of 32 had accidentally eaten peanut within the previous year, and only a quarter had succeeded in avoiding peanut entirely. When the result is an asthmatic episode, or a laryngeal reaction with a tight sensation in the throat, an adrenaline or bronchodilator inhaler may be sufficient but, if the child is not old enough to manage this, then family, friends and schoolteachers may need to be trained in first-aid measures. A pre-loaded adrenaline syringe may be kept available, and antihistamines and corticosteroids may also be needed. Arrangements should be considered so that access to medical help can be obtained if, at the time, there is no one available who can manage the injection, or if it fails to provide adequate relief.

At the time of starting school, a child requires extra care and, in the most severe cases, the teacher may be willing to look after an emergency kit and also keep special sweets in the classroom. The parents may have to explain what is required when a child stays for a school lunch, and the child may even learn to take spare food or a personal supply of sweets to avoid being isolated or penalized when other children are given something extra.

The insidious penalties for dietary error can be a particular problem in children with complex allergic conditions, including asthma and eczema. During trying times, there is no doubt that the part played by patient-support groups can be very helpful in severe cases. Fortunately, in the case of some food-intolerant reactions, for example, to egg and milk, there is a tendency for the condition to remit as the child gets older. From time to time, new foods may therefore be introduced tentatively, on a trial basis, under the supervision of a doctor or dietitian. In less severe cases, occasional indiscretions with small quantities of a poorly tolerated food may cause no harm, and the reintroduction of partially tolerated foods at intervals of a few days may provide a helpful way of re-establishing food tolerance.

THE DOCTOR-PATIENT RELATIONSHIP

Doctors who are aware of the fashionable trend towards the overdiagnosis of food allergy are sometimes sceptical in the face of genuine problems. Having seen many more problems caused by inappropriate dietary restriction than by true food allergy, doctors may sometimes insist on the reintroduction of poorly tolerated foods to the point where the patient may feel that it is difficult to obtain objective medical advice. It is therefore necessary to emphasize the importance, in cases of doubt, of an elimination diet and challenge tests. It is also important to emphasize the limited value of laboratory tests, except in coeliac disease and in the few cases where immediate food allergies can be identified through skin tests or laboratory tests for IgE antibodies.

In some instances, a patient with a disorder such as coeliac disease may be entirely unaware of the relevance of food to their symptoms. There is, therefore, a need for greater awareness among doctors of the problems which may require investigation, especially among patients who are intolerant to gluten and whose symptoms may not follow closely enough after the food is taken to allow recognition of the cause-and-effect relationship.

The tendency for patients to seek medical advice varies enormously from one condition to another. Those patients who correctly identify their own intolerance to one or two foods may take the appropriate avoidance measures and never see a doctor. Others who diagnose themselves or their children as having food intolerance in association with behavioural or psychologically based symptoms provide a much more complex problem. In some cases, the patient who presents this self-made diagnosis does not want or welcome the doctor's assessment. The consultation begins, not with a request for diagnosis, but with a request for help with the management of a restricted diet. In such cases, when carefully conducted tests give negative results, it must be accepted that some patients will nevertheless refuse to consider a diagnosis other than food allergy.

Food allergies have become a fashionable affliction, a substitution in some cases for the whimsical diagnoses of previous generations — including, in their time, 'dropped' stomach or kidneys, overprovided, redundant loops of bowel, vitamin imbalance, low blood sugar, and sucrose intolerance. Although fashions are once again changing, the trend towards diagnosing food intolerance or chronic candidiasis may divert attention from organic disease of another kind or from psychological problems that require other forms of treatment.

Nevertheless, without a sympathetic hearing, appropriate investigations, and much patience and support from their physicians, individuals who present with a fixed belief of their own illness will often lead limited disabled lives. They will seek confirmation of their self-diagnosis wherever they can, often resorting to 'black box' tests or 'black box' treatments. A few such patients, on investigation, may prove to have postinfectious conditions, such as the post-glandular fever syndrome (*Hamblin et al., 1983*; *Straus et al., 1985*), or other organic diseases. The majority of patients who present in this way have, however, a large psychiatric component to their ill health, which is likely to be denied as a possibility (see also p. 43).

DIAGNOSTIC TESTS

There has been a curious development, welcomed by some patients but heavily criticized by the medical profession, of the marketing of diagnostic tests which can be freely advertised regardless of their value and without any element of consumer protection. Patients who then realise that they have parted with their money for tests with no diagnostic use have, at present, no recourse. While biopsies of the small intestinal mucosa in patients with coeliac disease, and skin-prick tests or IgE-based laboratory tests in the diagnosis of immediate allergic reactions can be useful, these are very different from the large repertoire of diagnoses and treatments which have come to be based on unsubtantiated theories concerning food reactions.

The public should be warned against diagnostic tests which have not been validated and, indeed, against the dietary or other advice which may then be given on the basis of the inappropriate tests. Test methods which involve the placing of food drops under the tongue have been shown, in careful studies, to be valueless (*Lehman, 1980a*; *Royal College of Physicians, 1992*). After objective evaluation, skin tests that rely on the injection of different dilutions of the same material to find a 'neutralization point' have also been found to be useless (see Chapter 3). Other tests have depended on exposing a patient's blood to different food solutions and assessing how quickly the blood cells die — the so-called 'cytotoxic' test, which can be highly misleading (*Sethi et al., 1987*). Other inappropriate test methods have been used to incriminate *Candida* yeast infection as the cause of a wide range of vague symptoms, an accusation for which there is no sound evidence. Despite numerous attempts to assess these methods objectively, none of them can justify the prolonged and expensive treatment regimes that are often prescribed on the basis of such methods.

Other tests for food allergy are equally controversial. Commercial laboratories which advertise diagnostic tests may fail to distinguish between symptoms caused by an immunological reaction, for which useful tests are available, and those which have other causes and require a different diagnostic approach. The study referred to in Chapter 3 (*Sethi et al., 1987*) demonstrated that commercial laboratories which claim to diagnose food allergy often report widely discrepant results for pairs of blood or hair samples which are, in fact, taken from the same individual. In that particular study, non-existent allergies were also diagnosed in virtually all normal subjects and, in one case, dietary advice was given by post, based on the results of the blood test. In a situation that is beset with emotional overtones, it is all the more important that claims of this kind be looked at critically. A guide to allergy – what it is, how it is perceived, and how to approach the claims made about it – has now been published by the Royal College of Physicians of London (*1992*) and can be obtained from 11 St. Andrew's Place, London NW1 4LE.

THE NEED FOR BETTER INFORMATION

Patient-support groups can play an important part in providing the kind of detailed information that a physician may not always give, or may not be available to repeat and amplify. Parents of sick children may be especially grateful for the support which such societies provide. These societies depend especially on the kindness and personal involvement of public-spirited, caring people who may have experienced the same kind of illness within their own families. They themselves may often have felt isolated when trying to manage a difficult problem and therefore realise how helpful it is to have an opportunity to share experiences with others at local group meetings.

It should be noted that self-help groups may have both strengths and weaknesses. In food allergy and intolerance, as in other conditions which have attracted publicity, the provision of leaflets, booklets and personal advice concerning the medical or dietary management of a problem is only helpful if, in the first place, the diagnosis is correct. In the case of food allergy, the very real dangers of misdiagnosis have been outlined above. There is a need for the involvement of a physician who has sufficient objectivity to apply valid test methods in cases of doubt, while avoiding the use of unsubstantiated test methods. Enthusiasts are not always the best diagnosticians, and the public should be warned not only against the difficulties of self-diagnosis, but also against the random and wholesale diagnosis of food allergy as offered by commerical laboratories – and occasionally by doctors – on the basis of test methods which have no scientific basis.

In an attempt to diminish these hazards, some societies open their mailing lists only to those who have been medically diagnosed, for example, the Coeliac Society (P.O. Box 181, London NW2 2QY). Others have strong medical boards which provide policy advice, for example, the NVAS (Postbox 249, 3740 AE Baarn, The Netherlands), the British Allergy Foundation (St. Bartholomew's Hospital, West Smithfield, London EC1A 7BE) and the National Asthma Campaign (Providence Place, Upper Street, London N1). In recognizing the need to combine the commitment of volunteers and the help of experts, these organizations depend on the calibre of their medical advisers. At least of equal importance, as regards food intolerance, is the advice given by dietitians.

Most physicians now accept that their involvement with a patient cannot end with the issuing of a diagnosis and a prescription. They have therefore given their assistance in the setting up of patient-support groups. National specialist associations have also taken on the responsibility of issuing information leaflets on a number of topics. The American Academy of Allergy and Clinical Immunology has been exemplary in producing fact sheets. Australian and British societies (the British Allergy Foundation, the National Eczema Society, Australian Allergy Service, PO Box 946, N. Sydney, 2060) are not far behind.

Government agencies have contributed by issuing booklets such as *Look at the Label* (see Chapter 7), or in partnership with self-help groups – for example, when the Dutch Education Bureau of Food and Nutrition collaborated in the production of a food-intolerance databank. Non-governmental bodies have played their part. One of these is the Food and Drink Federation (6 Catherine Street, London WC2B 5JJ), which supplies a leaflet on food additives to anyone sending a stamped self-addressed envelope. They also supply physicians and dietitians with lists of food products that are free of ingredients, such as cow's milk, egg or colouring materials. DATA LIVO (P.O. Box 84185, 2508 AD The Hague, The Netherlands) also provides similar help.

Advice on food-intolerant reactions is helpful in a wide range of conditions, including coeliac disease, cow's milk reactions in infants, various types of food allergy, and intolerance caused by toxic substances, enzyme deficiencies, or the drug-like effects of substances such as caffeine. It is, therefore, important that the dissemination of current knowledge should not only encompass the facts, but also emphasize the point at which the facts are inconsistent with some of the more fashionable and fallacious opinions. Information by itself may not, however, be sufficient to counter some of the more entrenched views.

One of the problems which both medical and non-medical groups may fail to overcome is that of the self-diagnosed patients who insist that there is a connection, which they alone can identify, between a food or food additive and a specific symptom.

Much has been published concerning the relationship between foods and behavioural disorders. An obsession with this aspect in patients who show no evidence of such a connection can lead to the neglect of a psychiatric or other disease. This has been encouraged by repeatedly publicized suggestions that food colourings and preservatives carrying an E number are virtually the only cause of behavioural problems such as hyperactivity, aggressiveness, unmanageability, depression and listlessness. From the point of view of patient-support groups, the suspicion of a connection between nutrition and behaviour is a firm indication for investigation under medical supervision. Paradoxically, the anxieties concerning E numbers, which began with the 'man in the street' have now extended to more and more food manufacturers, who proudly proclaim the removal of additives from their products, even at the risk of increasing bacterial contamination.

While there is a need for more research to determine how far nutrition can affect behaviour, the publicity surrounding artificial additives as a possible cause of behavioural disorders has become a disadvantage. It is where this kind of publicity is most prominent that the fundamental problems of food allergy and food intolerance are most at risk of being dismissed or ridiculed. It is unwise to ignore the real problems caused by food intolerance, but it is equally unwise to cause unnecessary alarm.

CONCLUSION

The tendency to overdiagnose food-intolerant reactions has led to the mismanagement of a variety of other medical problems and neglect of illnesses which have been incorrectly labelled as a food allergy. Food reactions are, nevertheless, an important cause of ill health. Those who are themselves affected, or who have food-allergic children, can derive much help and comfort from patient-support groups and from the leaflets, booklets and personal advice now available from medical and lay organizations as well as from governmental departments.

Glossary

(including definitions contained in text)

Allergy: see p. 19

Amaranth red: see p. 129

Anaphylaxis: see p. 73

Angioedema: see p. 75

Anorexia: poor appetite

Antibody: see p. 59 and Fig. 4.5

Antibody, monoclonal: see p. 157; an artificially produced antibody produced by cells grown in a culture medium. The product of these cells can be designed to act as a highly specific chemical reagent

Antigen: a protein or other substance recognized by the body as 'foreign' and able to initiate an immune reaction

Arachidonic acid: a fatty acid released from phospholipids on the surface of mast cells and other cells, from which a number of powerful mediators are produced

Arrhythmia: irregular, abnormal heart beat rhythm

Atopic: liable to develop allergies

Autoantibody: an antibody which reacts with the body's own components

B cells: see p. 59

Bactericidal: capable of killing bacteria

Binge-eating: episodes of gorging

Biogenic amines: see p. 67

Brilliant blue: see p. 129

Brush-border enzymes: digestive enzymes attached to the surface (brush border) of the microvilli

Bulimia: disordered eating habits with episodes of binge-eating

Candida albicans: see p. 46

Candidiasis: infection by species of *Candida* yeast

Caramel: see p. 130; burnt sugar

Cellobiose: a disaccharide, formed from cellulose, which is sufficiently stable to avoid breakdown in the body

Challenge test: see pp. 87–8

Chemical hypersensitivity syndrome: see p. 35

Chronic urticaria: see p. 67

Cochineal: see p. 129

Coeliac disease: see p. 154

Complement: see pp. 59, 65

Corticosteroids: hormones (either synthetic or natural) with a basic structure similar to that of cortisone and which can be used as a drug or applied to the body surfaces to suppress inflammation temporarily

Dendrocyte: see p. 59

Dermatitis herpetiformis: see p. 165

Dimer: a chemical compound formed by the joining of two identical molecules

Disaccharidase: any enzyme which splits the two carbon rings of a disaccharide sugar

Diuretic: a substance which stimulates urine production

E numbers: see p. 126

Ecological illness: see p. 35

Eczema: see p. 79; a condition in which the skin (and especially the skin folds) can itch, redden, form crusts and weep fluid, especially after scratching

Enterocyte: see p. 53

Enteropathy: see p. 93

Environmental illness: see p. 35

Eosinophilia: see p. 40

Epidemiology: the study of disease in the community at large

Erythrosine: see p. 129

False food allergy: see p. 67

FEV$_1$: see p. 108

Food additive: see p. 123

Food allergy: see p. 19

Food aversion: see p. 20

Food intolerance: see p. 19

GALT: see p. 59

Gliadin: see p. 155

Gluten shock: see p. 163

Grandfather status: see p. 125

Gut-associated lymphoid tissue: see p. 59

Homeopathy: a theoretical approach to disease which depends on medicines that have some form of similarity to the organ affected and are used only in extremely dilute form

Humectants: see p. 128

Hydrolase: an enzyme which breaks down molecules by incorporating water into them (hydrolysis)

Hydrolysates: the products of hydrolysis

Hyperactivity: see p. 29

Hyperkinetic syndrome: see p. 30

Hyperventilation syndrome: see pp. 20, 50

Hypochromic: pale (usually applied to the appearance of red blood cells in iron deficiency anaemia)

Hypoglycaemia: low blood sugar

Hypolactasia: see p. 83

Ig: immunoglobulin

Immune reactions: see p. 19; reactions which are directed against 'foreign' substances which have entered the body

Immunodeficiency: impairment of the immune-complex reactions

Immunoglobulin: see Fig. 4.5

Immunoglobulins A, E, G, M: see pp. 60–1 and Fig. 4.5

Intrinsic factor: substance produced by the stomach which facilitates the absorption of vitamin B_{12}

Irritable bowel syndrome: see p. 71

Ketosis: acidosis; acidity of the body fluids

Ketotic diet: a diet which causes acidosis; used at one time to control childhood epilepsy

Leukotriene: substances which are synthesized from arachidonic acid (see also prostaglandins) by lipoxygenase enzymes

Lipase: see p. 56

Lymphatics: see p. 59

Lymphocyte: see p. 59

Lymphokine: see p. 65

Macrocytosis: see p. 163

Macrophage: see p. 59; a large scavenger cell which can destroy ingested particles, but can also act as an antigen-presenting cell and provoke an immune reaction; (dendritic cells can also do the same)

Maillard reaction: see p. 150

Mannitol: an unfermentable alcohol, used in metabolic studies to provide a stable molecule of small size, which can be traced as it passes through the body

Mast cell: a type of cell which is present below the surfaces and lining membranes of the body and can be triggered into releasing inflammatory substances, e.g. during the course of an allergic reaction

Metabolism: see p. 2

Methylisothiocyanate: a pesticide used in the wine industry to prevent secondary fermentation

Micelle: see p. 56

Microvilli: see p. 53

Monoclonal: see Antibody

Munchausen's disease: a disorder in which patients invent their symptoms or their disease, named after the mythical Baron Munchausen, whose stories defied belief

Myalgia: muscle pain

Nephrotic syndrome: see p. 114

Oral allergy syndrome: see p. 78

Osteomalacia: a condition in which bones become soft because of a deficiency of calcium or vitamin D (or both)

Osteoporosis: thin or brittle bones

Overactivity: see p. 30

Overnutrition: see p. 2

Papules: very small, raised areas of the skin

Peak flow meter: a simple measuring device used to check the breathing capacity of patients with any form of breathing difficulty

Pentamer: a chemical compound formed by the joining of five identical molcules

Peptidase: an enzyme capable of breaking down small proteins or peptides

Phenylketonuria: an inherited disease in which the body cannot metabolize due to a lack of a specific enzyme

Photochemical: involving the modification of a chemical effect on exposure to sunlight

Prolamins: see p. 154

Prostaglandins: substances synthesized from arachidonic acid by a variety of different cells which have powerful effects, notably by causing contraction or relaxation of smooth muscle (e.g. in blood vessels)

Proteases: see p. 56

Proteolytic: capable of breaking down protein

Pruritus: itching

Pseudoallergic reaction: see p. 67

Pulmonary haemosiderosis: a lung condition characterized by the deposition of iron in the tissues, usually derived from trivial, but repeated, bleeding

Reagin: see p. 73

Reticulin: see pp. 76, 158

Retort treatment: see p. 149

Rhinitis: a term loosely applied to any condition accompanied by a runny nose or sneezing

Scurvy: illness caused by a deficiency of vitamin C

Serotonin: see p. 110

Somatization: see p. 49

T cells: see p. 59

Tartrazine: see p. 129

Thrombocytopenia: see p. 114

Thrush: a condition in which there is a growth of yeast-like organisms in the mouth or genital regions

Toxins: substances which have a damaging or poisonous effect on living tissues

Urticaria: see p. 79

Vasodilatation: opening up of the blood vessels

Vesicles: blisters

Villi: see pp. 20, 53; a villus is a minute, finger-like projection from the mucous membrane of the small intestine which, together with the microvilli on its surface, adds enormously to the surface area in contact with any digested food passing through

Vitamin: (derived from 'vital amine'); a general name for a range of organic substances present in very small amounts in food, but serving an important function in the body's metabolism

Vitamin C: see p. 131

References

Acheson D. First report of the Advisory Group on the medical aspects of air pollution episodes – ozone. *Department of Health PL/CMO(19)7*, 7 May, 1991. *HMSO London*.

Akinyanju OO, Odusote KA. Cause of red soya syndrome is food dye orange-RN. *Lancet* 1983; ii: 1314.

Allen DH. Monosodium glutamate. In: *Food Allergy: Adverse Reactions to Food and Food Additives*. Metcalfe DD, Sampson HA, Simon RA, eds. Boston: Blackwell Scientific Publications, 1991, pp 261–6.

Allen DH, Delohery J, Baker FJ. Monosodium-*l*-glutamate-induced asthma. *J Allergy Clin Immunol* 1987; 80: 530–7.

Allen D, Delohery J. Metabisulphite induced asthma (abstr.) *J Allergy Clin Immunol* 1985; 75: 145.

Alun Jones VA. Irritable bowel syndrome. In: *Food and the Gut*. Hunter JO, Alun Jones V, eds. London: Baillière Tindall, 1985, 208–20.

Alun Jones VA, McLaughlin P, Shorthouse M, *et al*. Food intolerance: a major factor in the pathogenesis of irritable bowel syndrome. *Lancet* 1982; ii: 1115–7.

Ament MD, Rubin CE. Soy protein – another cause of flat intestinal lesion. *Gastroenterology* 1972; 62: 227–34.

American Academy of Allergy and Immunology Committee. *Adverse Reactions to Foods, 1984*. NIH Publication No. 84–2442, 1984.

American College of Physicians. Clinical ecology (position paper). *Ann Intern Med* 1989; 111: 168–78.

Amlot PL, Urbanek R, Youlten LJF, *et al*. Type 1 allergy to egg and milk proteins: comparison of 'skin-prick tests with nasal, buccal and gastric provocation test. *Int Arch Allergy Appl Immunol* 1985; 77: 171–3.

Anderson JW. Dietary fibre and diabetes. In: *Medical Aspects of Dietary Fibre*. Spiller GA, Kay RM, eds. London: Plenum Medical, 1980.

Anderson JA, Sogn DD, eds. Adverse food reactions that involve or are suspected of involving immune mechanisms: An anatomical characterization. In: *American Academy of Allergy and Immunology Committee on Adverse Reactions to Foods*. Washington, DC, NIAID, 1984, pp 43–102.

Andersson LB, Dreyfuss EM, Logan J, *et al*. Melon and banana sensitivity coincident with ragweed pollinosis. *J Allergy* 1970; 45: 310–9.

Anonymous. Coeliac disease. *Lancet* 1991; 337: 590.

Anonymous. Sumatriptain, serotonin, migraine, and money, *Lancet*, 1992; 339: 151–2.

Aslam M, Divas SS, Healy MA. Heavy metals in some Asian medicine and cosmetics. *Publ Hlth London* 1979; 93: 274–84.

Asslin J, Hebert J, Amlot J. Effects of in-vitro proteolysis on the allergenicity of major whey proteins. *J Food Sci* 1989; 54: 1037–9.

Association of County Councils Publications. *Additives in Food, Drink, Cosmetics and Medicines*. Association of County Councils, Eaton Sq, London, 1987.

Atherton DJ, Sewell M, Soothill JF, Wells RS. A double-blind, crossover trial of an antigen-avoidance diet in atopic eczema. *Lancet* 1978; i: 401–3.

Atkins FM, Steinberg SS, Metcalfe DD. Immediate adverse reactions to food in adults. II. A detailed analysis of reaction patterns during oral food challenge. *J Allergy Clin Immunol* 1985; 73: 356–63.

Bahna SL, Heiner DC. *Allergies to Milk*. New York: Grune & Stratton, 1980.

Baker GJ, Collett P, Allen DH. Bronchospasm induced by metabisulphite-containing foods and drugs. *Med J Aust* 1981; 71: 487–9.

Berrill WT, Eade OE, Fitzpatrick PF, Hyde I, MacLeod WM, Wright R. Bird-fancier's lung and jejunal villous atrophy. *Lancet* 1975; ii: 106–8.

Berry Brazelton T. *Toddlers and Parents*. London: Macmillan, 1976.

Bierman, CW, Shapiro GC, Christie DL, *et al*. Eczema, rickets, and food allergy. *J Allergy Clin Immunol* 1978, 61: 119–27.

Bjarnason I, Ward K, Peters TS. The leaky gut of alcoholism: Possible route of entry for toxic compounds. *Lancet* 1984: i: 179–81.

Black AP. A new diagnostic method in allergic disease. *Pediatrics* 1956; 17: 716–23.

Black DW, Rathe R, Goldstein RB. Environmental illness. A controlled study of 26 subjects with '20th century disease'. *JAMA* 1990; 264: 3166–70.

Blackwell B, Mabbitt LA. The tyramine content of cheese and its relationship to the hypertensive crisis after monoamine oxidase inhibition. *Lancet* 1965; i: 938–40.

Blackwell B, Marley E, Price J, Taylor D. Hypertensive interactions between monoamine oxidase inhibitors and foodstuffs. *Br J Psychiatr* 1967; 113: 349–65.

Bloom SR, Long RG, Polak JM. Hormones and the gastrointestinal tract. In: *Oxford Textbook of Medicine, 2nd Edition*. Weatherall DJ, Ledingham JGG, Warrell DA, eds. Oxford: Oxford Scientific, 1987, 12: 52–61.

Bock SA. Adverse reaction to foods during the first 3 years of life. *J Allergy Clin Immunol* 1985; 75: 178.

Bock SA. A critical evaluation of clinical trials in adverse reactions to food in children. *J Allergy Clin Immunol* 1986; 78: 165–74.

Bock SA, Atkins FM. The natural history of peanut allergy. *J Allergy Clin Immunol* 1989; 83: 900–4.

⋄ Bock SA, Lee WY, Remigio LK, May CD. Studies of hypersensitivity reactions to foods in infants and children. *J Allergy Clin Immunol* 1978; 62: 327–34.

Boughey HA. Bronchial hyperreactivity to sulphur dioxide: Physiologic and political implications. *J Allergy Clin Immunol* 1982; 69: 335–8.

Breneman JC, Metzler C, Hurst A, *et al*. Final report of the Food Allergy Committee of the American College of Allergists on the clinical evaluation of sublingual provocative testing method for diagnosis of food allergy. *Ann Allergy* 1974; 33: 164–6.

Brook CGD. Endocrinological control of growth at puberty. In: *Control of Growth*. Tanner JM, ed. London: Churchill Livingstone, 1981.

Buisseret PD. Common manifestations of cow's milk allergy in children. *Lancet* 1978; i: 304–5.

Buisseret PD, Youlton LJF, Heinzelmann DI, Lessof MH. Prostaglandin-synthesis inhibitors in prophylaxis of food intolerance. *Lancet* 1978; 1: 906–7.

Bullock RJ, Barnett D. Immunologic and clinical response to parenteral immunotherapy in peanut anaphylaxis: A case study using IgE and IgG4 immunoblot monitoring (In press).

Burge PS. Occupational asthma. In: *Respiratory Medicine*. Brewis RAL, Gibson GJ, Geddes EM, eds. London, Baillière Tindall, 1990, pp. 704–21.

Burke V, Kerry KR, Anderson CM. The relationship of dietary lactose refractory diarrhoea in infancy. *Aust Paediatr J* 1965; 1: 147–60.

Burkitt DP, Trowell HC. *Refined Carbohydrate Foods and Disease*. London: Academic Press, 1975.

Burr ML. Epidemiology. In: *Proceedings of the First Food Allergy Workshop*. Coombs RRA, ed. Oxford: Medical Education Service, 1980, 9–12.

Bush RK, Taylor SL, Busse W, *et al*. A critical evaluation of clinical trials in relation to sulfites. *J Allergy Clin Immunol* 1986; 78: 191–202.

Bush RK, Taylor SL, Nordlec JA, Busse WW. Soybean oil is not allergenic to soybean-sensitive individuals. *J Allergy Clin Immunol* 1985; 76: 242–5.

Caffrey EA, Sladen GE, Isaacs PET, Clark KGA. Thrombocytopenia caused by cow's milk. *Lancet* 1981; ii: 316.

Caldwell JH, Tennenbaum JI, Bronstein HA. Serum IgE in eosinophilic gastroenteritis. *N Engl J Med* 1975; 292: 1388–90.

California Medical Association Scientific Board Task Force on Clinical Ecology: Clinical Ecology – A critical appraisal [Information]. *Western Journal* 1986; 144: 239–45.

Caplin I. Report of the Committee on Provocative Food Testing. *Ann Allergy* 1973; 31: 375–81.

Cathebras P, Charmion S, Gonthier R, *et al*. Chronic fatigue, viruses and depression. *Lancet* 1991, 337: 564–5.

CDC Report. Outbreak of gastroenteritis due to copper poisoning. Vermont. *CMMWR* 1977; 26: 218–23.

Ceuppens JL, van Durmez P, Dooms-Goossens A. Latex allergy in patients with allergy to fruit. *Lancet* 1992; 339: 493.

Ciclitira PJ, Hunter JO, Lennox ES. Clinical testing of bread made from nullisomic 6A wheats in coeliac patients. *Lancet* 1980; ii: 234–5.

Cleave TL. *The Saccharine Disease.* Bristol: John Wright & Sons, 1974.

Clemmensen O, Hjorth N. Perioral contact urticaria from sorbic acid and benzoic acid in a salad dressing. *Contact Dermatitis*, 1982; 8: 1–6.

Coca AF. *Familial Non-Reaginic Food Allergy.* Springfield, IL: Charles C Thomas, 1942.

Condemi JJ. Unproved diagnostic and therapeutic techniques. In: *Food Allergy: Adverse Reactions to Food and Food Additives.* Metcalfe DD, Sampson HA, Simon RA, eds. Boston: Blackwell Scientific Publications, 1991, pp 392–404.

Conn EE. Cyanogenic glycosides. In: *Committee on Food Protection, Food and Nutrition Board, National Research Council, Report on: Toxicants Occurring Naturally in Foods.* Washington, DC: National Academy of Sciences, 1973, 299–308.

Cooke WT. Neurologic manifestations of malabsorption. In: *Handbook of Clinical Neurology.* Klawans HL, ed. Amsterdam, North Holland: 1976; 28: 225–41.

Cooke WT, Holmes FKT. Coeliac disease, inflammatory bowel disese and gluten intolerance. In: *Clinical Reactions to Food.* Lessof MH, ed. Chichester: John Wiley & Sons, 1983, 181–215.

Cooper BT, Holmes GKT, Ferguson R, Thompson RA, Allan RN, Cooke WT. Gluten-sensitive diarrhoea without evidence of coeliac disease. *Gastroenterology* 1980; 79: 801–6.

Crisp AH. Anorexia nervosa at normal body weight: The abnormal normal weight control syndrome. *Int J Psychiatr Med* 1981; 11: 203–33.

Crisp AH, McGuinness B. Jolly fat: the relationship between obesity and psychoneurosis in the general population. *BMJ* 1976; 1: 7–9.

Cronin E. *Contact Dermatitis.* Edinburgh: Churchill Livingstone, 1980.

Crook WG. *The Yeast Connection.* Jackson, TN: Professional Books, 1984.

Cummings NA, Vanden Bos GR. The twenty years Kaiser Permanente experience with psychotherapy and medical utilization. *Health Policy Quarterly* 1981; 1: 158–70.

Danna PL, Urban C, Bellin E, Rahal JJ. Role of candida in pathogenesis of antibiotic-associated diarrhoea in elderly inpatients. *Lancet* 1991; 337: 511–3.

Dannenberg F, Kessler HG. Application of reaction kinetics to the denaturation of whey proteins in heated milk. *Milchwissenschaft* 1988; 43: 3.

David TJ. Food additives. *Arch Dis Child* 1988; 63: 582–3.

David TJ. Reactions to dietary tartrazine. *Arch Dis Child* 1987; 62: 119–22.

David TJ, Waddington E, Stanton RHJ. Nutritional hazards of elimination diets in children. *Arch Dis Child* 1984; 59: 323–5.

Davidson GP, Townley RRW. Structural and functional abnormalities of the small intestine due to nutritional folic acid deficiency in infancy. *J Pediatr* 1977; 90: 590–4.

Denman AM. Allergy and joint complaints. In: *Allergy: An International Textbook.* Lessof MH, Lee TH, Kemeny DM, eds. Chichester: John Wiley & Sons, 1987, 565–76.

Denman AM, Mitchell B, Ansell BM. Joint complaints and food allergic disorders. *Ann Allergy* 1983; 51: 260–3.

de Weck AL. Pathophysiologic mechanisms of allergic and pseudoallergic reactions to foods, food additives and drugs. *Ann Allergy* 1984; 53: 583–6.

Dhivert H, Pyrpilis I, Joram C, et al. Etude comparée de trois extraits allergéniques de *Candida albicans* par la technique des tests cutanés, corrélation avec les taux d'IgE total et un RAST *Candida albicans*. *Bull Soc Franç Mycol Med* 1983; 12: 129–33.

DHSS. *Artificial Feeds for the Young Infant. Report No. 18*. London: HMSO, 1980.

Dicke WK. Coeliakie een onderzok naar de nadelige invloed van sommige graansoorten op de lijder aan coeliakie. (Doctoral thesis). University of Utrecht, Netherlands, 1950.

Dickey LD. *Clinical Ecology*. Springfield, IL: Charles C Thomas; 1976.

Dismukes WE, Wade JS, Lee JY, et al. A randomized, double-blind trial of nystatin therapy for the candidiasis hypersensitivity syndrome *N Engl J Med* 1990; 323: 1717–23.

Dohi M, Suko M, Sugiyama H, et al. Food-dependent exercise-induced anaphylaxis: A study on 11 Japanese cases. *J Allergy Clin Immunol* 1991; 87: 34–40.

Donovan GK, Torres-Pinedo R. Chronic diarrhoea and soy formulas. *Am J Dis Child* 1987; 41: 1069–74.

Donovan GR, Baldo BA. Cross-reactivity of IgE antibodies from sera of subjects allergic to both rye-grass pollen and wheat endosperm proteins: Evidence for common allergenic determinants. *Clin Exp Allergy* 1990; 20: 501–9.

Egger J, Carter CM, Graham PJ, et al. Controlled trial of oligoantigenic diet in the hyperkinetic syndrome. *Lancet* 1985; i: 540–5.

Egger J, Carter CM, Wilson J, et al. Is migraine food allergy? A double-blind controlled trial of oligoantigenic diet treatment. *Lancet* 1983; ii: 865–9.

Executive Committee of the American Academy of Allergy and Immunology. Candidiasis Hypersensitivity Syndrome. *J Allergy Clin Immunol* 1986; 78: 271–3.

Faux JA, Hendrick DJ, Anand BS. Precipitins to different avian serum antigens in bird-fancier's lung and coeliac disease. *Clin Allergy* 1978; 8: 101–8.

Feingold B. *Why Your Child is Hyperactive*. New York: Random House, 1975.

Feldman JM, Histaminuria from histamine-rich foods. *Arch Intern Med* 1984; 143: 2099–2102.

Fell, P, Brostoff J. A single dose desensitisation for summer hay fever. *Eur J Clin Pharmacol* 1990; 38: 77–9.

Ferguson R, Holmes GKT, Cooke WT. Coeliac disease, fertility and pregnancy. *Scand J Gastroenterol* 1982; 17: 65–8.

Finn R, Cohen HN. Food allergy: Fact or fiction? *Lancet* 1978; i: 426–8.

Firer MA, Hopkins CS, Hill DJ. Possible role for rotavirus in the development of cow's milk enteropathy in infants. *Clin Allergy* 1988; 18: 53–61.

Food Labelling Regulations 1984. SI 1984/1305. London: HMSO, 1984.

Franz MJ. Figuring fast food. *Diabetes Forecast*. November, 1987, 49–50.

Freeman IJ. Aspects of hyperventilation in cardiology. *Cardiol Pract* 1989; 7: 20–5.

Frei P. Changing habits in food and drug reactions. In: *Progress in Allergy and Clinical Immunology*. Pichler WJ, Stadler BM, Dahinden CA, et al., eds. Toronto: Hografe and Huber, 1989, 471–7.

Friberg L, Olesen J, Iversen HK, Sperling B. Migraine pain associated with middle cerebral artery dilatation: Reversal by sumatriptan. *Lancet* 1991; 338: 13–7.

Friedman RA, Doyle WJ, Casselbrant ML, et al. Immunologic-mediated eustachian tube obstruction: a double-blind crossover study *J Allergy Clin Immunol* 1983; 71: 442–7.

Fries JH. Studies on the allergenicity of soybean. *Ann Allergy* 1971; 29: 1–5.

Galloway JH, Marsh ID, Bittiner SB, *et al.* Chinese herbs for eczema, the active compound? *Lancet* 1991; 337: 566.

Garriga MM, Bjerkebile C, Metcalfe DD. A combined single-blind, double-blind, placebo-controlled study to determine the reproducibility of hypersensitivity reactions to aspartame. *J Allergy Clin Immunol* 1991; 87: 821–7.

Garrow J, Blaza S. Energy requirements in human beings. In: *Human Nutrition*. Neuberger A, Jukes TH, eds. Lancaster: MTP Press, 1982, 1–21.

Gee S. On the coeliac affection. *St. Bartholomew's Hosp Rep* 1888; 24: 17–20.

Gern JE, Yang EY, Evrard HM, *et al.* Allergic reactions to milk-containing "dairy free" products (Abstr.). *J Allergy Clin Immunol* 1990; 85: 273.

Gershwin ME, Ough C, Bock A, *et al.* Grand rounds: Adverse reactions to wine. *J Allergy Clin Immunol* 1985; 75: 411–20.

Gibson A, Clancy R. Management of chronic idiopathic urticaria by the identification and exclusion of dietary factors. *Clin Allergy* 1980; 10: 699–704.

Goldberg DP, Cooper B, Eastwood MP, *et al.* A standardised psychiatric interview for use in community surveys. *Br J Prevent Soc Med* 1970; 24: 18–23.

Goldman AS, Anderson DW Jr, Sellers WA, *et al.* Milk allergy. I. Oral challenge with mild and isolated milk proteins in allergic children. *Pediatrics* 1963; 32: 425–43.

Goodman MD, McDonnell JT, Nelson HS, *et al.* Chronic urticaria exacerbated by antioxidant food preservatives, butylated hydroxyanisole (BHA) and butylated hydroxytoluene (BHT). *J Allergy Clin Immunol* 1990; 86: 570–5.

Gryboski JD, Katz J, Reynolds D, Herskovic T. Gluten intolerance following cow's milk sensitivity: two cases with coproantibodies to milk and wheat protein. *Ann Allergy* 1968; 26: 33–6.

Gumowski PI, Lech B, Chaves I, Girard JP. Chronic asthma and rhinitis due to *Candida albicans, Epidermophyton* and *Trichophyton*. *Ann Allergy* 1987; 59: 48–51.

Haffejee IE. The pathophysiology, clinical features and management of rotavirus diarrhoea. *Quart J Med* 1991; 79: 289–99.

Hager C, Faber J, Daczuni A, *et al.* Prevalence of postenteritis cow's milk protein intolerance. *Israel J Med Sci* 1987; 23: 1128–31.

Hall MA, Lanchbury JSS, Bolsover WJ, *et al.* HLA association with dermatitis herpetiformis is accounted for by a *cis*- or *trans*-associated DQ heterodimer. *Gut* 1991; 32: 487–90.

Halmepuro L, Bjorksten F. Immunological partial identity between pollen and food allergens. *Allergy* 1985; 3: 70–1.

Hamblin TJ, Hussain J, Akbar AN *et al.* Immunological reason for chronic ill health after infectious mononucleosis. *BMJ* 1983; 287: 85–8.

Hanington E. Migraine. In: *Clinical Reactions to Food*. Lessof MH, ed. Chichester: John Wiley & Sons, 1983, 155–80.

Hanington E, Lessof MH. Allergy. In: *Migraine*. Blau JN, ed. London: Chapman & Hall, 1987, 355–66.

Hannaway PJ, Hopper GDK. Severe anaphylaxis and drug-induced beta-blockade. *N Engl J Med* 1983; 308: 1536.

REFERENCES

Hansen LG, Host A, Osterballe O. Allergic reactions to unhomogenised milk and raw milk. *Ugeskr Laeger* 1987; 149: 909–11.

Harada S, Agarwal DP, Goedde HW, *et al.* Possible protective role against alcoholism for aldehyde dehydrogenase iso-enzyme deficiency in Japan. *Lancet* 1982; ii: 827.

Harley JP, Matthews CG, Eichman C. Synthetic food colors and hyperactivity in children: A double-blind challenge experiment. *Pediatrics* 1978; 62: 975–83.

Harley JP, Ray RS, Thomas L, *et al.* Hyperkinesis and food additives: Testing the Feingold hypothesis. *Pediatrics* 1978; 61: 818–28.

Harries MG, Parkes PEG, Lessof MH, Orr STC. Role of bronchial irritant receptors in asthma. *Lancet* 1981; i: 5–7.

Harrison M, Kilby A, Walker Smith JA, *et al.* Cow's milk protein intolerance: A possible association with gastroenteritis, lactose intolerance, and IgA deficiency. *BMJ* 1976; 1: 1501–4.

Harvey RF, Salih SW, Read AW. Organic and functional disorders in 2000 gastroenterology out-patients. *Lancet* 1983; i: 632–4.

Hawkins RC. Meal/snack frequencies of college students: A narrative study. *Behav Psychother* 1979; 7: 85–9.

Heatley RV, Denburg JA, Bayer N, Bienenstock J. Increased plasma histamine levels in migraine patients. *Clin Allergy* 1982; 12: 145–9.

Hekkens WTJM. The evolution in research in prolamin toxicity: from bread to peptide. In: Food Allergy and Food Intolerance. Somogyi JC, Müller HR, Ockhuisen T, eds. *Bibl Nutr Dieta.* Basel: Karger, 1991; 48: 90–104.

Herxheimer H. The skin sensitivity to flour of bakers' apprentices: a final report of long term investigation. *Acta Allergol* 1967; 28: 42–9.

Hill DJ, Firer MA, Shelton MJ, Hoskins CS. Manifestations of milk allergy in infancy: Clinical and immunological findings. *J Paediatr* 1986; 109: 270–6.

Hirsch SR, Kalbfleisch JH, Golbert TM, *et al.* Rinkel injection therapy: A multicentre controlled study. *J Allergy Clin Immunol* 1981; 68: 133–55.

Holmes GKT, Prior P, Lane MR, *et al.* Malignancy in coeliac disease – Effect of a gluten-free diet. *Gut* 1989; 30: 333–8.

Host A, Halken S. A prospective study of cow's milk allergy in Danish infants during the first 3 years of life. Clinical course in relation to clinical and immunological type of hypersensitivity reaction. *Allergy* 1990; 45: 487–96.

Host A, Samuelsson EG. Allergic reactions to raw, pasteurised and homogenised/pasteurised cow's milk: A comparison. *Allergy* 1988; 43: 113–8.

Hughes M, Clark N, Forbes L, Colin-Jones DG. A case of scurvy. *BMJ* 1986; 293: 366.

Hunter JO. Provocation testing and food sensitivity *N Engl J Med* 1991; 325: 1172.

Hyams JS, Krause PJ, Gleason PA. Lactose malabsorption following rotavirus infection in young children. *J Pediatr* 1981; 99: 916–8.

Iyngkaran N, Abidin S, Meng LL, Yadav M. Egg protein-induced villous atrophy. *J Pediatr Gastroenterol Nutr* 1982; 1: 29–33.

Iyngkaran N, Davis K, Robinson MJ, *et al.* Cow's milk protein-sensitive enteropathy. An important contributing cause of secondary sugar intolerance in young infants with acute infective enteritis. *Arch Dis Child* 1979; 54: 39–43.

Iyngkaran N, Robinson MJ, Prathap R, *et al.* Cow's milk protein sensitive enteropathy. Combined clinical and histological criteria for diagnosis. *Arch Dis Child* 1978; 53: 20–6.

Iyngkaran N, Yadav M, Looi LM, *et al*. Effect of soy protein on the small bowel mucosa of young infants recovering from acute gastroenteritis. *J Paediatr Gastroenterol Nutr* 1988; 7: 68–75.

Jacobsen DW. Adverse reactions to benzoates and parabens. In: *Food allergy: Adverse Reactions to Foods and Food Additives*. Metcalfe DD, Sampson HA, Simon RA, eds. Boston: Blackwell Scientific Publications, 1991, 276–87.

James P, Ralph A. What is a healthy diet? *Med Int* 1990; 82: 3364–8.

Jansen TLTA, Wagenaar CGJ, Mulder CJJ. Coeliac disease and lymphoma. *Lancet* 1991; 338: 318.

Jenkins HR, Pincott JR, Soothill JE, *et al*. Food allergy: The major cause of infantile colitis. *Arch Dis Child* 1984; 59: 326–9.

Jewett DL, Fein G, Greenberg MH. A double-blind study of symptom provocation to determine food sensitivity. *N Engl J Med* 1990; 323: 429–33.

Jost R, Fritsché R, Pahud JJ. Reduction of milk protein allergenicity through processing. *Bibl Nutr Dieta*. Basel: Karger, 1991; 48: 127–37.

Jost R, Monti JC, Pahud JJ. Whey protein allergenicity and its reduction by technological means. *Food Technol* 1987; 41: 118–21.

Kaufman LD, Gruber BL, Gregerson PK. Clinical follow-up and immunogenetic studies of 32 patients with eosinophilia-myalgia syndrome. *Lancet* 1991; 337: 1071–4.

Keating MV, Jones RT, Worley NJ, *et al*. Immunoassay of peanut allergens in food-processing materials and finished foods. *J Allergy Clin Immunol* 1990; 86: 41–4.

Kemeny DM, Price JF, Richardson V, *et al*. The IgE and IgG subclass antibody response to foods in babies during the first year of life and their relationship to feeding regimen and the development of food allergy. *J Allergy Clin Immunol* 1991; 87: 920–9.

Kemeny DM, Urbanek R, Amlot PL, *et al*. The subclass of IgG in allergic disease. 1. IgG subclass antibodies in immediate and non-immediate food allergy. *Clin Allergy* 1986; 16: 571–82.

Kenyon JN. Diagnostic techniques using bioenergetic recording methods: The science of bioenergetic regulatory medicine. *Am J Acupunct* 1986; 14: 5–15.

Kerr GR, Wu-Lee M, El-Lozy M, McGandy R, Stare FJ. In: *Glutamic Acid: Advances in Biochemistry and Physiology*. Filer LJ, Garattini S, Kare MR, Reynolds WA, eds. New York: Raven Press, 1979, 375.

Kerr GR, Wu-Lee M, El-Lozy M, McGandy R, Stare FJ. Objectivity of food symptomatology surveys. Questionnaire on the 'Chinese Restaurant Syndrome'. *J Am Dietetic Assoc* 1977; 71: 263–8.

Kidd III JM, Cohen SH, Sosman AJ, Fink JN. Food-dependent exercise-induced anaphylaxis. *J Allergy Clin Immunol* 1983; 71: 407–11.

Kilbourne EM, Rigan-Perez JG, Heath CW Jr, *et al*. Clinical epidemiology of toxic-oil syndrome: Manifestations of a new illness. *N Engl J Med* 1983; 309: 1408–14.

King MB, Mezey G. Eating behaviour of male racing jockeys. *Psychol Med* 1987; 17: 249–53.

Kleijnen J, ter Riet G, Knipschild P. Acupuncture and asthma: A review of controlled trials. *Thorax* 1991; 46: 799–802; 788–97 (*editorial*).

Klein NC, Hargrove RL, Slesinger MH, Jeffries GH. Eosinophilic gastroenteritis. *Medicine (Baltimore)* 1970; 49: 299–319.

Kleinman RE. Milk protein enteropathy after acute infectious gastroenteritis: Experimental and clinical observations. *J Pediatr* 1991; 118: 5111–5.

Koepke J, Chrostopher K, Chai H, Selner J. Dose-dependent bronchospasm from sulfites in isoetharine. *JAMA* 1984; 251: 2982–3.

Koerner CD, Sampson HA. Diets and Nutrition. In: *Food Allergy: Adverse Reactions to Food and Food Additives*. Metcalfe DD, Sampson HA, Simon RA, eds. Boston: Blackwell Scientific Publications, 1991, 332–54.

Kosnai, I, Kuitunen P, Siimes MA. Iron deficiency in children with coeliac disease on treatment with gluten-free diet. Role of intestinal blood loss. *Arch Dis Child* 1979; 54: 375–8.

Kuitunen P, Viskorpi JK, Savilahti E, Pelkonen P. Malabsorption syndrome with cow's milk intolerance. Clinical findings and course in 54 cases. *Arch Dis Child* 1975; 50: 351–6.

Kulczycki A Jr. Aspartame-induced urticaria. *Ann Intern Med* 1986; 104: 207–8.

Kwok RHM. Chinese restaurant syndrome. *N Engl J Med* 1968; 278: 796.

Labib M, Gama R, Wright J, *et al*. Dietary maladvice as a cause of hypothyroidism and short stature. *BMJ* 1989; 298: 232–3.

Lacey JH. The patient's attitude to food. In: *Clinical Reactions to Food*. Lessof MH, ed. Chichester: John Wiley & Sons, 1983, 35–58.

Lacey JH, Chadband C, Crisp AH, *et al*. Variation in energy intake of adolescent girls. *J Hum Nutr* 1978; 32: 419–26.

Lake AM. Food protein-induced gastroenteropathy in infants and children. In: *Food Allergy: Adverse Reactions to Food and Food Additivies*. Metcalfe DD, Sampson HA, Simon RA, eds. Boston: Blackwell Scientific Publications, 1991, 173–85.

Lauritzen M, Olesen J. Leao's spreading depression. In: *Migraine*. Blau JN, ed. London: Chapman & Hall, 1987, 387–402.

Lavaud F, Cossart C, Reiter V, *et al*. Latex allergy in patient allergic to fruit. *Lancet* 1992; 339: 492–3.

Lawton R. Goat's milk. In: *Health Hazards of Milk*. Freed D, ed. London: Baillière Tindall, 1984, 150–6.

Lee DA, Winslow NR, Speight AND, Hey EN. Prevalence and spectrum of asthma in childhood. *BMJ* 1983; 286: 1256–8.

Lee TH, Hoover RL, Williams JD, *et al*. Dietary enrichment with eicosapentaenoic and decosahexaenoic acids in human subjects impairs in vitro neutrophil and monocyte function and leukotriene generation. *N Engl J Med* 1985; 312: 1217–24.

Leeming RJ, Blair JA. Serum crithidia levels in disease. *Biochem Med* 1980; 23: 122–5.

Lehman CW. A double-blind study of sublingual provocative food testing: A study of its efficacy. *Ann Allergy* 1980a; 45: 144–9.

Lehman CW. The leukocytic food allergy test: A study of its reliability and reproducibility. Effect of diet and sublingual food drops on this test. *Ann Allergy* 1980b; 45: 150.

Lessof MH. Adverse reactions to food additives. *J R Coll Phys* 1987; 21: 237–40.

Lessof MH, Gant V, Hinuma K, *et al.* Recurrent urticaria and reduced diamine oxidase activity. *Clin Exp Allergy* 1990; 20: 373–6.

Lessof MH, Kemeny DM, Price JF. IgG antibodies to food in health and disease. *Allergy Proc* 1991; 12: 305–7.

Lessof MH, Wraith DG, Merrett TG, Merrett J, Buisseret PD. Food allergy and intolerance in 100 patients – local and systemic effects. *Quart J Med* 1980; 195: 259–71.

Levine AS, Labuza TP, Morley JE. Food technology: A primer for physicians. *N Engl J Med* 1985; 312: 628–34.

Levitt MD, Bereggren T, Hastings J, Bond JH. Hydrogen (H_2) catabolism in the colon of the rat. *J Lab Clin Med* 1974; 84: 163–7.

Levitt MD, Lasser RB, Schwartz JS, Bond JH. Studies of flatulent patients. *N Engl J Med* 1976; 295: 260–2.

Lloyd AR, Hickie I, Boughton CR, *et al.* The prevalence of chronic fatigue syndrome in an Australian population. *Med J Aust* 1990; 153: 522–8.

Lloyd-Still JD. Chronic diarrhoea of childhood and the misuse of elimination diets. *J Pediatr* 1979; 95: 10–13.

Lockey SD. Allergenic reactions due to FD+C yellow number 5 tartrazine, an aniline dye used as a colouring agent in various steroids. *Ann Allergy* 1959; 17: 719–21.

Lucas ML, Cooper BT, Lei FH, *et al.* Acid microclimate in coeliac and Crohn's disease: A model for folate malabsorption. *Gut* 1978; 19: 735–42.

Lum LC. Hyperventilation and anxiety state. *Proc R Soc Med* 1981; 74: 1–4.

Macdonald I. Nutrition in the Western World. In: *Clinical Reactions to Food.* Lessof MH, ed. Chichester: John Wiley, 1983, 1–14.

MacGregor FB, Abernethy VE, Dahabra S, *et al.* Hepatotoxicity to herbal remedies. *BMJ* 1989; 299: 1156–7.

Mackarness R. *Chemical Victims.* London: Pan Books, 1980.

Mackarness R. *Not All in the Mind.* London: Pan Books, 1976.

MacNair A. New dietary reference values. *BMJ* 1991; 303: 520–1.

MAFF Working Party. *Food Surveillance, Paper No. 18. London: HMSO, 1987.*

Maga JA. Amines in food. CRTC Crit Rev Food Sci Nutr 1978; 10: 373–403.

Magarian GJ. Hyperventilatory syndromes: Infrequently recognised common expressions of anxiety and stress. *Medicine (Baltimore)* 1982; 61: 219–36.

Maki M, Hallstrom O, Marttiners A. Reaction of human non-collagenous polypeptides with coeliac disease autoantibodies. *Lancet* 1991; 338: 724–5.

Malhotra SL. A comparison of unrefined wheat and rice diets in the management of duodenal ulcer. *Postgrad Med J* 1978; 54: 6–9.

Mansfield LE, Bowers CH. Systemic reaction to papain in a non-occupational setting. *J Allergy Clin Immunol* 1983; 71: 371–4.

Mansfield LE, Vaughan TR, Waller SF, *et al.* Food allergy and adult migraine: Double-blind and mediator confirmation of allergic etiology. *Ann Allergy* 1985; 55: 126–9.

Mansfield LE, Ting S, Haverly RW, Yoo TJ. The incidence and clinical implications of hypersensitivity to papain in an allergic population confirmed by blinded oral challenge. *Ann Allergy* 1985; 55: 541–3.

Marsh MN. Immunocytes, enterocytes and the lamina propria: An immunological framework of coeliac disease. *J R Coll Phys* 1983; 17: 205–12.

Mattes JA, Gittelman R. Effects of artificial food colorings in children with hyperactive symptoms. A critical review and results of a controlled study. *Arch Gen Psychiatr* 1981; 38: 714–8.

Maulitz RM, Pratt DS, Schocket AL. Exercise-induced anaphylactic reaction to shellfish. *J Allergy Clin Immunol* 1979; 63: 433–4.

Maxwell JD. Liver disorders associated with dietary constituents. In: *Food and the Gut*. Hunter JO, Alun Jones V, eds. London: Baillière Tindall, 1985, 288–302.

May CD. Food allergy – Material and ethereal. *N Engl J Med* 1980; 302: 1142–3.

Mazza DS, O'Sullivan M, Grieco MH. HIV-1 infection complicated by food allergy and allergic gastroenteritis: A case report. *Ann Allergy 1991*; 66: 436–40.

McKeigue PM. Relation of central obesity and insulin resistance with higher diabetes prevalence and cardiovascular risk in South Asians. *Lancet* 1991; 337: 382–6.

McMillan SA, Haughton DJ, Biggart JD, *et al*. Predictive value for coeliac disease of antibodies to gliadin, endomysium and jejunum in patients attending for jejunal biopsy. *BMJ* 1991; 303: 1163–5.

Meara RH. Skin reactions in atopic eczema. *Br J Dermatol* 1965; 67: 60–4.

Mechamic D, Kleinman A. Ambulatory medical care in the People's Republic of China. *Am J Pub Health* 1980; 70: 62–6.

Miskelly FG, Burr ML, Vaughan-Williams E, *et al*. Infant feeding and allergy. *Arch Dis Child* 1988; 63: 388–93.

Mitchell-Heggs CAW, Conway M, Cassar J. Herbal medicine as a cause of combined lead and arsenic poisoning. *Hum Exp Toxicol* 1990; 9: 195–6.

Molfino NA, Wright SC, Katz I, *et al*. Effect of low concentrations of ozone on inhaled allergen responses in asthmatic subjects. *Lancet* 1991; 338: 199–203.

Moneret-Vautrin DA. False food allergies: Non-specific reactions to foodstuffs. In: *Clinical Reactions to Food*. Lessof MH, eds. Chichester: John Wiley & Sons, 1983, 135–53.

Moneret-Vautrin DA. Biogenic amines. *Bibl Nutr Dieta*. Basel: Karger 1991; 48: 61–71.

Moneret-Vautrin DA, Einhorn C, Tisserand J. Le role du nitrite de sodium dans les urticaires histaminique d'origine alimentaire. *Ann Nutr Alim* 1980; 34: 1125–32.

Moneret-Vautrin DA, Hatahet R, Kanny G, Ait-Djafer Z. Allergenic peanut oil in milk formulas. *Lancet* 1991; 338: 1149.

Muir P, Nicholson F, Banatvala JE, Bingley PJ. Coxsackie B virus and postviral fatigue syndrome. *BMJ* 1991; 302: 658–9.

Munro IC. The ingredients of food: How they are tested and why they are selected. *J Allergy Clin Immunol* 1986; 78: 133–9.

Murdoch RD, Pollock I, Young E, Lessof MH. Food additive-induced urticaria: Studies of mediator release during provocation tests. *J R Coll Phys* 1987; 21: 262–6.

Murphy M. Somatization: Embodying the problem. *BMJ* 1989; 298: 1331–2.

Mylotte M, Egan-Mitchell B, McCarthy CF, McNicholl B. Coeliac disease in the West of Ireland. *BMJ* 1973; 3: 498–9.

Nanda R, James R, Smith H, *et al.* Food intolerance and the irritable bowel syndrome. *Gut* 1989; 30: 1099–1104.

Nelson TL, Klein GL, Galant SP. Severe eosinophilic gastroenteritis successfully treated with an elemental diet (Abstr). *J Allergy Clin Immunol* 1979; 63: 198.

Newman Taylor AJ. Occupational Allergy. In: *Allergy: An International Textbook.* Chichester: John Wiley & Sons; 1987: 359–80.

Niphadkar PV, Patil SP, Bapat MM. Legumes, the most important food allergen in India (Abstr). *Proc Eur Acad Allergy*, 1992.

Nixon PGF. 'Total allergy syndrome' or fluctuating hypocarbia. *Lancet* 1982; i: 404.

Noone C, Menzies IS, Banatvala JE, Scopes JW. Intestinal permeability and lactose hydrolysis in human rotaviral gastroenteritis assessed simultaneously by non-invasive differential sugar permeation. *Eur J Clin Invest* 1986; 16: 217–25.

Nylander I. The feeling of being fat and dieting in a school population: An epidemiologic interview investigation. *Acta Socio-Med Scand* 1971; 3: 17–26.

O'Driscoll BRC, Milburn HJ, Kemeny DM, Cochrane GM, Panayi GS. Atopy and rheumatoid arthritis. *Clin Allergy* 1985; 15: 547–53.

O'Neil CE, Lehrer SB. Occupational Reactions to Food Allergens. In: *Food Allergy: Adverse reactions to Food and Food Additives.* Metcalfe DD, Sampson HA, Simon RA, eds. Boston: Blackwell Scientific Publications, 1991, 207–36.

Olson GB, Kanaan MN, Gersuk GM, *et al.* Correlation between allergy and persistant Epstein-Barr virus infections in chronic-active Epstein-Barr virus-infected patients. *J Allergy Clin Immunol* 1986a; 78: 308–314.

Olson GB, Kanaan MN, Kelly LM, Jones JF. Specific allergen-induced chronic-active Epstein-Barr virus infections. *J Allergy Clin Immunol* 1986b; 78: 315–20.

Ornish D, Brown SE, Scherwitz LW, *et al.* Can lifestyle changes reverse coronary artery disease? *Lancet* 1990; 336: 129–33.

Paganelli R, Levinsky RJ, Atherton DJ. Detection of specific antigen within circulating immune complexes: Validation of the assay and its application to food antigen-antibody complexes formed in healthy and food-allergic subjects. *Clin Exp Immunol* 1981; 46: 44–53.

Paganelli R, Levinsky RJ, Brostoff J, Wraith DG. Immune complexes containing food proteins in normal and atopic subjects after oral challenge and effect of sodium cromoglycate on antigen absorption. *Lancet* 1979; i: 1270–2.

Palmer RL. The dietary chaos syndrome: A useful new term? *Br J Med Psychol* 1979; 52: 187–90.

Panush RS, Food-induced ("allergic") arthritis: Clinical and serological studies. *J Rheumatol* 1990, 17, 291–4.

Panush RS, Stroud RM, Webster EM. Food-induced (allergic) arthritis: Inflammatory arthritis aggravated by milk. *Arthr Rheum* 1986; 29: 220–6.

Papageorgiou N, Lee TH, Nagakura T, Wraith DG, Kay AB. Neutrophil chemotactic activity in milk-induced asthma. *J Allergy Clin Immunol* 1983; 72: 75–83.

Parke AL, Hughes GRV. Rheumatoid arthritis and food: A case study. *BMJ* 1981; 282: 2027–9.

Parsons DS. Mechanisms of absorption. In: *Oxford Textbook of Medicine, 2nd Edition*. Weatherall DJ, Ledingham JGG, Warrell DA, eds. Oxford: Oxford University Press 1987; 12: 92–8.

Parsons LG. Coeliac disease. *Am J Dis Child* 1932; 43: 1293–346.

Pastorello E, Ortolani C, Luraghi M, *et al.* Evaluation of allergy etiology in perennial rhinitis. *Ann Allergy* 1985; 55: 854–6.

Pelikan Z, Pelikan-Filpek M. Bronchial response to the food ingestion challenge. *Ann Allergy* 1987; 58: 164–72.

Penn RG. Adverse reactions to herbal medicines. *Adverse Drug React Bull* 1983; 102: 376–9.

Penn RG. Adverse reactions to herbal and other unorthodox medicines. In: *Iatrogenic Diseases*. D'Arcy PF, Griffin JP, eds. Oxford: Oxford University Press, 1986, 898–918.

Peskett SA, Platts-Mills TAE, Ansell BM, Stearnes GM. Incidence of atopy in rheumatic diseases. *J Rheumatol* 1981; 8: 321–4.

Pollock I, Warner JO. A follow-up study of childhood food additive intolerance. *J R Coll Phys* 1987; 21: 248–50.

Pollock I, Warner JO. Effect of artificial colours on childhood behaviour. *Arch Dis Child* 1990; 65: 74–7.

Popham P, *A Poisoned City*, Independent on Sunday Magazine, 11 May 1991, 26–33.

Prausnitz C, Küstner H. Studien uber die Uberemfindlichkeit. *Zentralbl Bakteriol Orig* 1921; 86: 160–9.

Price JF. Paediatric Allergy. In: *Allergy: An International Textbook*. Lessof MH, Lee TH, Kemeny DM, eds. Chichester: John Wiley & Sons, 1987, 423–53.

Price SF, Smithson KW, Castell DO. Food sensitivity in reflux oesophagitis. *Gastroenterology* 1978; 75: 240–3.

Raffle PAB, Lee WR, McCallum RI, Murray R. *Hunter's Diseases of Occupations*, London: Hodder and Stoughton, 1987, pp 251, 309.

Rapoport JL, Effects of dietary substance in children. *J Psychiatr Res* 1982–3; 17: 187–91.

Reilly DT, Taylor MA, McSharry C, Aitchison T. Is homeopathy a placebo response? Controlled trial of homeopathic potency, with pollen in hayfever as model. *Lancet* 1986; 2: 881–6.

Reiman H–J, Ring J, Ultsch B, Wendt P. Intragastral provocation under endoscopic control (IPEC) in food allergy: Mast cell and histamine changes in gastric mucosa. *Clin Allergy* 1985; 15: 195–202.

Reports of the Scientific Committee for Food (12th Series). EUR 7823. British Library Loan 3828, 4F, 1982.

Reunala T, Blomqvist K, Tarpila S, *et al.* Gluten-free diet in dermatitis herpetiformis. I. Clinical response of skin lesions in 81 patients. *Br J Dermatol* 1977; 97: 473–80.

Rinkel HJ, Randolph TGY, Zeller M. *Food Allergy*. Springfield, IL: Charles C. Thomas, 1951.

Rippere V. Food additives and hyperactive children: A critique of Conners. *Br J Clin Psych* 1983; 22: 19–32.

Rix KJB, Pearson DJ, Bentley SJ. A psychiatric study of patients with supposed food allergy. *Br J Psychiatr* 1984; 145: 121–6.

Robertson CF, Heycock E, Bishop J, *et al.* Prevalence of asthma in Melbourne schoolchildren: Changes over 26 yers. *BMJ* 1991; 302: 1116–8.

Robertson DA, Ayres RC, Smith CL, Wright R. Adverse consequences arising from misdiagnosis of food allergy. *BMJ* 1988; 297: 719–20.

Rowe KS. Synthetic food colourings and 'hyperactivity': A double-blind crossover study. *Aust Paediatr J* 1988; 24: 143–7.

Royal College of Physicians. *Allergy – Conventional and Alternative Concepts.* London: Pitman Medical, 1992.

Royal College of Physicians. *Medical Aspects of Dietary Fibre. London:* Pitman Medical, 1980.

Sampson HA. Role of immediate food sensitivity in the pathogenesis of atopic dermatitis. *J Allergy Clin Immunol* 1983; 71: 473–80.

Sandler M, Youdim MBH, Hanington E. A clinical and biochemical correlation between tyramine and migraine. *Headache* 1970; 10–12: 43–51.

Savilahti E. Cow's milk allergy. *Allergy* 1981; 36: 73–88.

Scadding GK, Brostoff J. Low-dose sublingual therapy in patients with allergic rhinitis due to house dust mite. *Clin Allergy* 1986; 16: 483–91.

Schaumberg HH, Byck R, Gerstl R, Marshman JH. Monsodium-glutamate: Its pharmacology and role in the Chinese restaurant syndrome. *Science* 1969; 163: 826–8.

Selner JC, Standenmayer H. Food allergy: Psychological considerations. In: *Food Allergy: Adverse Reactions to Food and Food Additives.* Metcalfe DD, Sampson HA, Simon RA, eds. Boston: Blackwell Scientific Publications, 1991, pp 370–81.

Seixas FA. Medications, drugs and alcohol. In: *Fermented Food Beverages in Nutrition.* Gastineau CF, Darby WJ, Turner TB, eds. New York, Academic Press, 1979, pp 245–56.

Sessa A, Desiderio A, Perin A. Effect of acute ethanol administration on diamine oxidase activity in the upper gastrointestinal tract of the rat. *Alcoholism: Clin Exp Res* 1984; 8: 185–90.

Sethi TJ, Lessof MH, Kemeny DM, *et al.* How reliable are commercial allergy tests? *Lancet* 1987; i: 92–4.

Settipane GA, Chafee FH, Postman M, *et al.* Significance of tartrazine sensitivity in chronic urticaria of unknown aetiology. *J Allergy Clin Immunol* 1976; 57: 541–6.

Sheldon W. Coeliac disease: A relation between dietary starch and fat absorption. *Arch Dis Child* 1949; 24: 81–7.

Shenassa MM, Perelmutter L, Gerrard JW. Desensitisation to peanut. (Abstr). *J Allergy Clin Immunol* 1985; 75: 177.

Shenkin A. Trace element and vitamin deficiency. *Med Int* 1990; 82: 3397–401.

Simon RA. Adverse reaction to food and drug additives. In: *Progress in Allergy and Clinical Immunology.* Pichler WJ, Stadler BM, Dahinden CE, eds. Toronto: Hografe and Huber, 1989, 467–70.

Skipworth M. M & S victim of international wine scandal. *The Sunday Times* 1992 Feb 16: I, 5.

Sloan AE, Powers ME. A perspective on popular perceptions of adverse reactions to food. *J Allergy Clin Immunol* 1986; 78: 127–33.

Smith SJ, Markandu ND, Rotellar C, Elder DM, MacGregor GA. A new or old Chinese restaurant syndrome? *BMJ* 1982; 285: 1205.

Smith MR, Morrow T, Safford RJ. The role of food additives and intolerance reactions to food. *Bibl Nutr Dieta*. Basel: Karger 1991; 48: 72–80.

Stead RH, Perdue MH, Blennerhasset MG, *et al*. The innervation of mast cells. In: *The Neurocrine-Immune Network*. Boca Raton, FL: CRC Press, 1989, pp 19–37.

Stevenson DD, Simon RA. Sensitivity to ingested metabisulfites in asthmatic subjects. *J Allergy Clin Immunol* 1981; 68: 26–32.

Stevenson DD, Simon RA, Lumry WR, Mathison DA. Adverse reactions to tartrazine. *J Allergy Clin Immunol* 1986; 78: 182–91.

Stewart DE. Emotional disorders misdiagnosed as physical illness: Environmental hypersensitivity, candidiasis hypersensitivity, and chronic fatigue syndrome. *Int J Ment Health* 1990; 3: 56–68.

Straus SE, Tosato G, Armstrong G, *et al*. Persistent illness and fatigue in adults with evidence of Epstein-Barr virus infection. *Ann Intern Med* 1985; 102: 7–16.

Strobel S, Brydon WG, Ferguson A. Cellobiose/mannitol sugar permeability test complements biopsy histopathology in clinical investigation of the jejunum. *Gut* 1984; 25: 1241–6.

Sturgess RP, Macartney JC, Makgoba MW, *et al*. Differential up-regulation of intercellular adhesion molecule-1 in coeliac disease. *Clin Exp Immunol* 1990; 82: 489–92.

Swinson CM, Levi AJ. Is coeliac disease underdiagnosed? *BMJ* 1980; 281: 1258–60.

Tabuenca JM. Toxic-allergic syndrome caused by ingestion of rapeseed oil denatured with aniline. *Lancet* 1981; ii: 567–8.

Taylor B, Wadsworth J, Wadsworth MEJ, Beckham CS. Changes in the reported prevalence of childhood eczema since the 1939–45 war. *Lancet* 1984; ii: 1255–7.

Taylor J, Busse WW, Sachs MI, *et al*. Peanut oil is not allergenic to peanut-sensitive individuals. *J Allergy Clin Immunol* 1981; 68: 372–5.

Taylor SL, Bush RK, Selner JC, *et al*. Sensitivity to sulfited foods among sulfite-sensitive subjects with asthma. *J Allergy Clin Immunol* 1988; 81: 1159–67.

Thiel H, Ulmer WNT. Baker's asthma: Development and possibility of treatment. *Chest* 1980; 78 (suppl): 400–5.

Thompson WG, Heaton KW. Functional bowel disorders in apparently healthy people. *Gastroenterology* 1980; 79: 283–8.

Tobi M, Morag A, Ravid Z, *et al*. Prolonged atypical illness associated with Epstein-Barr virus infection. *Lancet* 1982; i: 61–4.

Towns SJ, Mellis CM. Role of acetyl salicylic acid and sodium metabisulfite in chronic childhood asthma. *Pediatrics* 1984; 73: 631–7.

Trewby PN, Chipping PM, Palmer SJ, *et al*. Splenic atrophy in adult coeliac disease: Is it reversible? *Gut* 1981; 22: 628–32.

Turner KJ. Epidemiology of atopic disease. In: *Allergy: An International Textbook*. Lessof MH, Lee TH, Kemeny DM, eds. Chichester: John Wiley & Sons, 1987, 337–46.

Tylleskar T, Barea M, Bikangi N, *et al*. Cassava cyanogens and konzo, an upper motorneurone disease found in Africa. *Lancet* 1992; 339: 208–11.

van der Kamer JH, Wijers HA, Dicke WK. Coeliac disease. IV. An investigation into the injurious constituents of wheat in connection with their action on patients with coeliac disease. *Acta Paediatr Scand* 1953; 42: 223–31.

van Metre TE. Unproven procedures for diagnosis and treatment of food allergy. *NER Allergy Proc* 1987; 8: 17–21.

Vaughan TR, Mansfield LE. Neurological reactions to food and food additives. In: *Food Allergy: Adverse Reactions to Food and Food Additives*. Metcalfe, DD, Sampson HA, Simon RA, eds. Boston: Blackwell Scientific Publications 1991, pp 355–69.

Veien NK, Haltel T, Justesen O, Nørholm A. Oral challenge with balsam of Peru. *Contact Dermatitis* 1985; 12: 104–7.

Vicario JL, Serrano-Rios M, San Andres F, Arnaiz-Villena A. HLA-DR3, DR4 increase in chronic stage of Spanish oil disease. *Lancet* 1982; i: 276.

Vitoria JC, Camarero C, Sojo A, *et al*. Enteropathy related to fish, rice and chicken. *Arch Dis Child* 1982; 57: 44–8.

Wadsworth M. Inter-generational differences in child health. In: *Measuring Sociodemographic Change*. OPCS occasional paper. London: OHMS, 1985, 34: 51–8.

Walker WA. Antigen handling by the small intestine. *Clin Gastroenterol* 1986; 15: 1–20.

Walker Smith JA. Cow's milk intolerance as a cause of post-enteritis diarrhoea. *J Paediatr Gastroenterol Nutr* 1982; 1: 163–6.

Walker Smith JA. Milk intolerance in children. *Clin Allergy* 1986; 16: 183–90.

Walsh BJ, Baldo BA, Bass DJ, *et al*. Insoluble and soluble allergens from wheat grain and wheat dust: Detection of IgE binding in inhalant and ingestion allergy. *NER Allergy Proc* 1987; 8: 27–33.

Warner JO, Hathaway MJ. Allergic form of Meadow's syndrome (Munchausen by proxy). *Arch Dis Child* 1984; 59: 151–6.

Wattrich B, Stager J, Johansson SG. Celery allergy associated with birch and mugwort pollinosis. *Allergy* 1990; 45: 466–76.

Whitfield MF, Barr DGD. Cow's milk allergy in the syndrome of thrombocytopenia with absent radius. *Arch Dis Child* 1976; 51: 337–43.

WHO. Study Group Report on Diet, Nutrition, and Prevention of Communicable Diseases. Geneva: WHO, 1990.

Williams DG. Allergy and the kidney. In: *Allergy: An International Textbook*. Lessof MH, Lee TH, Kemeny DM, eds. Chichester: John Wiley & Sons, 1987, 553–63.

Wilson NM. Food-related asthma: A difference between two ethnic groups. *Arch Dis Child* 1984; 59: 84–7.

Wilson NM, Silverman M. The diagnosis of food sensitivity in childhood asthma. *J R Soc Med* 1985; 78 (suppl 5): 11–16.

Wilson N, Scott A. Double-blind assessment of additive intolerance in children using a 12–day challenge period at home. *Clin Allergy* 1989; 19: 267–72.

Wilson N, Vickers H, Taylor G, Silverman M. Objective test for food sensitivity in asthmatic children: Increased bronchial reactivity after cola drinks. *BMJ* 1982; 284: 1226–8.

Wolf SI, Nicklas RA. Sulfite sensitivity in a seven-year-old child. *Ann Allergy* 1985; 54: 420–3.

Wraith DG. Respiratory diseases. In: *Proceedings of the First Food Allergy Workshop*. Coombs RRA, ed. Oxford: Medical Education Services, 1980, 64–8.

Young E, Patel S, Stoneham M, *et al*. The prevalence of reactions to food additives in a survey population. *J R Coll Phys* 1987; 21: 241–7.

Zeiger RS, Heller S, Mellor MH, *et al*. Effect of combined material and infant food-allergen avoidance on development of atopy in early infancy: A randomised study. *J Allergy Clin Immunol* 1989; 84: 72–89.

Zioudrou C, Streaty RA, Klee WA. Opioid peptides derived from food proteins. The exorphins. *J Biol Chem* 1979; 254: 2446–9.

Zwetchkenbaum JF, Skufca R, Nelson HS. An examination of food hypersensitivity as a cause of increased bronchial responsiveness to inhaled methacholine. *J Allergy Clin Immunol* 1991; 88: 360–4.

Index

acetic acid 130
acquired immunodeficiency syndrome
  (AIDS) 105
acupuncture 47, 49–50
additive 10, 33
  food 10, 21, 32, 36, 70
adrenaline 68, 94, 121, 146, 164
adverse reaction, management of 117
aflatoxin 14
agar 131
albumin, in milk 143
alcohol 67–8, 70, 84, 107–8, 133
  and migraine 108
aldehyde dehydrogenase 84
aldolase 40, 84
allergen 143
allergy 65
  remission rate 99
almond, cyanogens in 136
alternative medicine 35–6, 43
aluminium 145
amaranth red 129
amine 67, 69, 106, 110, 164
  biogenic 21
amphotericin 46
anaemia 94, 103
  hypochromic 162

anaphylactic response 75
anaphylaxis 73, 94, 102–3
  exercise–induced 102
  fruit 121
  milk 121
  mustard 121
  nuts 121
  sesame seed 121
  spices 121
angioedema 75, 94
  and eosinophilia 105
annatto 129
anorexia nervosa 25–6
antibiotic 85
antibody 55, 74, 144
  anti-EMA 158, 161
  antigliadin 158, 161
  antireticulin 157–8, 161, 166
anticaking agent 125, 131
antifoaming agent 125
antigen 58, 66, 98
antioxidant 83, 124–5, 131, 135
aphthous stomatitis 163
arginine 151
arrhythmia 31
arthritis 112
  rheumatoid 113

ascorbic acid 126
aspartame 133, 135
aspirin 103, 118
astaxanthin 129
asthma 37–8, 93, 96, 131
   adult 108
   and eosinophilia 105
   food-induced 97
   occupational 38, 115
   potentiating factor 97
   prevalence 96
atheroma 5
atmospheric pollution 37
autoantibody 158, 161
autonomic nervous system 55
azo colour 32

B cell 59
bacterial fermentation 71, 85
bactericidal agent 83
baker's asthma 115
balsam 135
banana 101
barley 155
beans 68, 101
   and migraine 109
   cyanogens in 136
   lectins in 136
bed-wetting 9
beef 146
beer 128
benzoate 126–7, 130, 133
benzoic acid 125, 130
berries 82, 91
betaphenylethylamine 69
bile 56
bile salts 53
binge eating 22
biogenic amine 67
bird-fancier's lung 108
bleacher 125
bran 11
brassica 136
bread 128
breath hydrogen 21

breath hydrogen test 88, 105
breathlessness 9
bromelain 125
bronchodilator 118
brush-border enzymes 53
buffalo milk 144
bulimia 22, 24, 26
bulking agent 125
butylated hydroxyanisole 126, 131, 133, 135
butylated hydroxytoluene 131, 133, 135

cabbage 82
cadaverine 69
caffeine 31, 82–3, 103
calciferol 165
calcium 7, 117, 142, 145, 173
calcium propionate 124, 128
Candida 46, 146
candidiasis 9, 175
cantaxanthin 129
caramel 10, 126, 130
caraway 135
carbohydrate 12
carotene 130, 144
carrageenan 131
casein 142–4, 148–9, 152
   hydrolysate 96
   protease-digested 151
casein hydrolysate 151–2
cassava 81–2
catecholamine 68
celery 78, 101
   psoralens in 136
cellobiose 76
cereal 91, 155–6
challenge test 20, 88, 97
cheese 67–8, 128
   and migraine 108
   mozzarella 129, 144
cheese ripening 150
chemical hypersensitivity syndrome 35
chestnut 101
chicken 79, 93

Chinese Restaurant Syndrome 139
chlorophyll 10, 129
chocolate 68, 91
  and migraine 109
cholesterol 16
chromium 7
chymotrypsin 151
cinnamon 135
citric acid 126
citrus fruit 68–9, 105
claret 128
clinical ecology 35, 43
coal-tar dye 133–4
cochineal 129
coeliac disease 19, 75–6, 78, 91, 154
  prevalence 159
coeliac society 170
coffee 31, 68, 105
cola 31, 97
colitis 94
  cow's milk 106
colophony 38
colour 32, 129
colouring 125
complement 59, 65
contact dermatitis 117, 133
contamination 139
copper 7, 39, 128–9
coronary artery disease 3, 14
corticosteroid 48, 94, 118, 121
  eczema 118
cow's milk 78–9, 85, 89, 91, 93, 142
  allergy 94
  and colitis 106
  and urticaria 106
  intolerance 103
  nephrotic syndrome 114
cow's milk-protein intolerance 91
cream 68
Crohn's disease 106
cromolyns 118
cross-sensitization 100
cucumber 82
cyanide 82
cyanogen 136
cyanogenic glycoside 81

cystic fibrosis 103
cytotoxic food test 45

dairy product 68, 146
databank 140
deafness 98
defect, enzyme 83
deficiency, enzyme 81, 83
dementia 164
dendrocyte 59
depression 48, 68, 164
dermatitis, contact 117
dermatitis herpetiformis 165
diabetes 3–4, 12, 161
diagnosis 87
diamine 68, 107
diamine oxidase 69, 107
diarrhoea 94, 164
  fatty 103–4, 161
  gluten-sensitive 100
diet
  elimination 118
  exclusion 118, 120
  maternal 146
dietary allowance, recommended
  (RDAs) 169
digestion 52
dinoflagellate 82
disaccharidase 164
disaccharide sugar 92
disodium cromoglycate 118
diuretic 83
diverticulitis 12
dodecyl gallate 131
dopamine 164
Down's syndrome 161
drug residue 124
drugs, beta-blocking 103
dust
  flour 38
  grain 38

E number 126, 178–9
eating disorder 24

ecological illness 35
eczema 38, 47, 79, 82, 85, 107,
        117–8, 135, 146–7
    egg 121
    infantile 95
    prevention 95
egg 78, 85, 89, 91, 93, 97, 105, 107,
        125, 140, 168, 174
    and migraine 109
    and urticaria 106
    eczema 121
    nephrotic syndrome 114
egg allergy 77
elimination diet 118
emulsifier 125, 166
enterocyte 53, 58, 92
enteropathy 93
environment 38
environmental control unit 41, 45
environmental illness 35, 47
enzyme 19, 52–3, 55–6, 70
    angiotensin-converting 158
    brush-border 158
    proteolytic 38
enzyme deficiency 81, 83, 92, 138
eosinophilia 40, 105
eosinophilia-myalgia syndrome 40
eosinophilic gastroenteritis 105
epidemiology 20
epilepsy 31, 112
epinephrine 121
epoxy resin 38
erythrosine 127, 129
esterase 53
exclusion diet 118, 120

false food allergy 67
fat 2, 4, 6, 25, 99
fat deposition 24–5
fatigue 9
fatigue syndrome 43
fatty acid 93, 142, 144
fermentation 128, 148
FEV$_1$ 108
fibre 6–7, 11, 16

fish 67–8, 73, 78–9, 87, 89, 91, 93,
        97, 108, 168
    and migraine 109
    and urticaria 106
    nephrotic syndrome 114
fish oil 15
fits 164
flavour modifier 125
flavour-enhancing agent 131
flavouring 124, 135–6
flour 100–1
flour dust 38
fluoride 7
folic acid 163, 165
food, occupational reaction to 115
food additive 10, 21, 32, 36, 70,
        123–4
food allergy 19, 29, 80, 88, 175
food antigen 58, 99
food aversion 20
food colour 140
food faddism 22, 24
food intolerance 52, 80–1, 90, 100
    diagnosis 19, 88
    residue 71, 85
food labelling 10, 140, 171
free fatty acid 56
freezant 126
fructose 84, 128
fruit 100
    anaphylaxis 121
    citrus 68–9, 105
fungus 81

gallstone 103
galvanized container 39
gastrin 53
gastroenteritis 92, 137, 146, 152
gastrointestinal infection 91
giardiasis 104
gliadin 76, 155–6
glucose 128
glutamic acid 131
glutamine 155
glutemin 156

gluten 78, 91, 93, 140, 155–6
   intolerance 21
   sensitivity 154
   shock 163
gluten-free 166
glycerol 131
glycoalkaloid 81
goat's milk 118, 144
gout 113
grain dust 38
'grandfather' status 125
grape 103
grape products 168
guar gum 12–3
gum 131
gut-associated lymphoid tissue
   (GALT) 59

hair test 45
headache 9, 108
heart disease 4, 14
heat denaturation 150
herbal remedies 48
herring 68
histamine 67–9, 107, 112
histidine 67
homoeopathy 49
homogenization 148
hordein 156
hormones 55, 69
Howell-Jolly body 162
humectant 128
hydrogen 85, 105
hydrolysate 118, 147
hydrolysate, casein 96
   milk 96
hydroxytoluene 126
hyperactivity 9, 29–31
hyperkinetic syndrome 30
hypersensitivity, delayed 107
hypersensitivity pneumonitis 78, 116
hyperventilation 20, 42, 50, 84
hypnosis 47
hypoglycaemia 69, 84

hypolactasia 81, 83
   secondary 104

IgA deficiency 161
IgE-mediated reaction 75, 102
IgG
   antibody 93
   subclasses 76
immune complex 75
immune reaction 74
immune-complex reaction 77
immunity, mucosal 58
immunodeficiency 46
immunoglobulin 59
   in milk 143
immunoglobulin A (IgA) 60, 78
immunoglobulin E (IgE) 61, 74, 93
immunoglobulin M (IgM) 60
improver 125
infantile fit 142
infection, intestinal 103
   virus 159
infertility 164
insomnia 9
intestinal infection 85
intestinal motility 70
intestinal permeability 76, 137
intolerance, additive 33
   cow's milk 103
   cow's milk-protein 91
   protein 31
intrinsic factor 53
iodine 7, 145
iron 7, 142, 145
irritable bowel 71, 83, 85
isocyanate 38
isomaltase 53

joint symptoms 112–3
juniper 135

kefir 150
ketoconazole 46

ketotic diet 112
kidney 114
killer cell 65
kinesiology 48

L-tryptophan 40
lactalbumin 143
lactase 53, 71, 83, 92, 143, 166
lactic acid 83
lactic fermentation 150
Lactobacillus 150
lactoglobulin 143
lactose intolerance 21, 143, 164
lactose tolerance test 104
lead 129
lecithin 125–6
lectin 136, 157
legume 82
lentil 101
leukotriene 15, 61
lignin 12
lima bean 81
lipase 53, 56, 93
liquorice 82
lovage 135
lymphatic system 59
lymphocyte 59
    intraepithelial 93
lymphokine 65
lysine 151

mackerel 81
macrocytosis 163
macrophage 59
magnesium 7, 164
Maillard reaction 150
maize 155
malabsorption 58
malnutrition 25
maltase 92
manganese 7
mannitol 76
mast cell 60–1, 67
maternal diet 146
meat 68

melon 101
menstruation 24–5
mercuric sulphide 129
metabisulphite 82
metabolism 2–5
metabolize 2
methionine 145
methylenedianiline 39
methyltransferase 69, 107
metronidazole 85
micelle 56
microfold cell 59
microvilli 53, 92
migraine 32, 68, 108
    and foods 109
milk 68, 97, 101, 105, 140, 168, 174
    anaphylaxis 121
    buffalo 144
    cow's 78–9, 85, 89, 91, 93, 142
    different types of 145
    fermented 150
    goat's 118, 144
    hydrolysate 96
    sheep's 118
    soya 94
milk fermentation 150
milk formula 151
milk processing 148
milk substitute 146
millet 81
molybdenum 7
monoamine 68
monoamine oxidase 68
monoclonal antibody 157, 166
monoglyceride 56
monosodium glutamate 131, 133,
    137–8
mozzarella cheese 129, 144
mucoprotein 69
mucosa 58
mucosal damage 164
mucous glycoprotein 55
Munchausen's disease 90, 169
mustard 78, 168
    anaphylaxis 121
myalgia 40

myalgic encephalomyelitis (ME) 43

nephrotic syndrome 114
  and foods 114
neurological symptoms 108
neutralizing dose 44
nitrate 130, 133
noradrenaline 164
nuts 78, 89, 91, 97, 101, 168
  anaphylaxis 121
  and migraine 109
nystatin 46

oats 155
obesity 3, 23, 25, 27
obstruction 98
occupational asthma 108
octopamine 69
octyl gallate 131
olive 128
onion 68
oral allergy syndrome 78
orange 106
orange-RN 138
osteomalacia 165
osteoporosis 165
otitis media, serous 98
overactivity 30
overbreathing 42
overnutrition 2
oxalic acid 126, 136
ozone 37

palpitation 9
papain 125, 138
paprika 130
paraben 133
parsley, psoralens in 136
pasteurization 148–9
pea 101
peak flow meter 108
peanut 14, 66, 91, 173
peanut oil 148

peas, psoralens in 136
pectin 12–3
pepsin 52, 125, 151
pepsinogen 52
peptidase 53, 164
permeability, intestinal 76
pesticide 124
Peyer's patches 59, 98
pharmacological reaction 82
phenylketonuria 31
phosphate 142
photochemical pollution 37
phytate 13, 145
pickling 128
placebo 21
plasticizer 41
platelet 163
platinum salt 38
pollution 36, 38
  atmospheric 36–7
  photochemical 37
pork 67–8
  nephrotic syndrome 114
post-glandular fever syndrome 175
potassium 164
preservative 5, 124–5, 130, 140
prevalence 138
processed food 140
proctitis 94
prolamin 155–6
proline 155
propionate 131
propionic acid 83, 130
propylene glycol 128
prostaglandin 61, 68, 105
protease 56
protein 6, 142, 155–6
protein hydrolysate 147, 166, 173
protein intolerance 31
proteolytic enzyme 135
provocation-neutralization test 44
pruritus 70
pseudoallergic reaction 67, 80–1
psoralen 136
psychiatric illness 28
pulmonary haemosiderosis 95

pulse test 44
putresceine 69

radioallergosorbent test (RAST) 89
raffinose 12
rapeseed oil 40
reaction, pharmacological 82
    pseudoallergic 138
    skin 106
reagin 73
red bean 82
resin 135
reticulin 76
retort treatment 149
rhinitis 93–4, 98
    occupational 115
rhubarb 136
riboflavin 142
rice 11, 79, 93, 155
rotavirus 92
rye 155

salt 16
sauerkraut 67
sausage 67
schizophrenia 28, 164
scombroid fish 81
scurvy 25
seafood 68
secalin 156
selenium 7
self-help 170
serotonin 110
sesame seed, anaphylaxis 121
sesame seeds 168
sheep's milk 118
shellfish 82, 103, 168
skin test 89, 106
smog, industrial 38
sneezing 98
sodium chloride 128
sodium metabisulphite 10, 39, 108,
    128, 133
sodium nitrate 124

sodium nitrite 70, 83, 135
sodium stearyl-lactylate 128
solvent 125, 131
somatization 49
sorbate 127
sorbic acid 124–5, 130
sorbitol 126, 131
soya 78–9, 91, 93, 96, 100–1, 118,
    145, 168
soya milk 94, 145
soybean 82, 125, 145
spearmint 135
spices 168
    anaphylaxis 121
splenic atrophy 163
stabilizer 125
stachyose 12
starch 12, 128
stearyl-lactylate 131
storage protein (prolamin) 154
strawberry 106
stress 69
sublingual test 44
sucrase 53, 92
sucrose 128
sugar reaction 30
sulphite 39, 124, 126, 131, 140
sulphiting agent 130–1
sulphur dioxide 37, 39, 82, 102, 108,
    130, 133, 138, 140
sunset yellow 127, 129
suppressor T cell 66
sweetener 125
synephrine 69

T cell 59, 165
tangerine 105
target cell 163
tartrazine 31, 126–7, 129, 134, 137
tea 68, 105
tenderizer 135
test
    breath-hydrogen 105
    intradermal 89
    lactose tolerance 104

test (*continued*)
  radioallergosorbent (RAST) 89
  skin-prick 106
thickener 166
thrombocytopenia 114
thrush 46, 146
tin 39
tinnitus 9
titanium oxides 126, 129
tolerance 66, 98
total allergy 23
toxic-allergic syndrome 40
toxic-oil syndrome 40
toxin 81, 88, 140, 145
transglutaminase 158
tricresyl phosphate 39
trypsin 125, 151
tumeric 126
tuna 81
turnip 82
type 1 reaction 74
type 2 reaction 76
type 3 reaction 77
type 4 reaction 78
tyramine 67–8, 70
tyrosine 67, 164

UHT heating 149
ulcer, mouth 163
ulcerative colitis 106
uric acid 114
urticaria 32–3, 67, 69, 75, 79, 82–3,
    106, 117, 135
  and cow's milk 106
  and eosinophilia 105
  chronic, and benzoate 133

egg 106
fish 106

vanilla 105, 135
Vega machine 48
vegan diet 170
vegetable 105
villi 20–1, 53, 76, 78–9, 161, 163
villous atrophy 93
vinegar 128
viral infection 43, 159
vitamin deficiency 117
vitamins 7–8, 16, 145, 173
vitamin A 144
vitamin B_{12} 165
vitamin C 126, 131, 142, 145
vitamin D 142, 164–5
vomiting 73, 94

wheat 11, 91, 100–1, 103, 105, 155,
    168
wheat starch 156
whey 142, 148–9, 151–2
white flour 11
wine 39, 69, 108, 128, 133
wine vinegar 168

yeast 68, 128
yoghurt 104, 150

zein 156
zinc 7, 142, 164